Capacity-building and Pandemics

Jun Jie Woo

Capacity-building and Pandemics

Singapore's Response to Covid-19

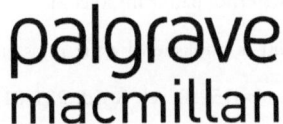

Jun Jie Woo
National University of Singapore
Singapore, Singapore

ISBN 978-981-15-9452-6   ISBN 978-981-15-9453-3   (eBook)
https://doi.org/10.1007/978-981-15-9453-3

This Palgrave Macmillan imprint is published by the registered company Springer Nature Singapore Pte Ltd.
The registered company address is: 152 Beach Road, #21-01/04 Gateway East, Singapore 189721, Singapore

For Debbie and Harvey

PREFACE

Singapore's early success in managing the Covid-19 pandemic has received much attention from researchers and observers from across the world. A study by the T.H. Chan School of Public Health at Harvard University had even described Singapore's early efforts to detect and contain the Covid-19 coronavirus as the 'gold standard of near-perfect detection'. Yet despite these accolades and its reputation as a leading medical hub, Singapore also experienced high rates of Covid-19 infections. These were fuelled by large infection clusters that had emerged in Singapore's migrant worker dormitories.

This book provides a policy-oriented understanding of the institutional drivers and processes that have underpinned Singapore's response to Covid-19 pandemic. It focuses specifically on the policy capacities that have been built up after the SARS crisis and how these have been translated into policy responses during the Covid-19 pandemic. It will also discuss the capacity shortcomings or deficiencies that may have created the aforementioned policy blind-spots. In doing so, this book aims to provide a deeper understanding of how policy capacity can be built up and mobilised in response to a policy crisis.

While much has been said about the epidemiological aspects and healthcare implications of the Covid-19 pandemic, there remains insufficient research and analysis on the institutional and policy bases of successful Covid-19 responses and interventions. By taking a policy capacity approach to understanding Singapore's Covid-19 response, this book will provide both policy scholars and practitioners with a useful analytical framework through which pandemic policy responses can be understood and evaluated.

Singapore   Jun Jie Woo

Acknowledgements

Every book is a labour of love. This book would not have been possible without the love and support of my wife Debbie and my son Harvey. All that I do is for the two of you.

Given that the bulk of this book was written during Singapore's 'Circuit Breaker' period, its pages are infused with the joy, laughter and frustrations of family life amidst a global pandemic.

In the process of writing this book, I have benefited immensely from the support and advice of friends, mentors and colleagues.

These include Leong Ching, M. Ramesh, Giliberto Capano, Benjamin Cashore, Kris Hartley, Christopher Tan, Benjamin Low, Lucas Neo and Cheryl Song. I am also thankful to the IPS community for their support and guidance, specifically Gillian Koh and Christopher Gee.

August 2020   Jun Jie Woo

CONTENTS

Contents

LIST OF TABLES

CHAPTER 1

Introduction

Abstract This chapter will provide a broad introduction to the topics that will be covered in the rest of this book and present a brief overview of Singapore's political, economic and policy context, focusing in particular on its public administration and policy processes. Particular attention will be paid to Singapore's healthcare system. A brief outline of the proceeding chapters will also be included in this chapter. This introductory chapter will therefore serve as a 'roadmap' for the rest of the book.

Keywords Covid-19 · Singapore · Policy capacity · Singapore governance

The Covid-19 pandemic has given rise to significant, social, economic and public health implications for Singapore. As of writing, the number of confirmed Covid-19 infections in Singapore has exceeded 55,000 while 27 people have passed away due to complications arising from the coronavirus. The rapid rise in Covid-19 infections had also prompted the Singapore government to implement a "circuit breaker" on 7 April 2020. The circuit breaker acted as a de facto lock down by placing restrictions on social and economic activities.

J. J. Woo, *Capacity-building and Pandemics*,
https://doi.org/10.1007/978-981-15-9453-3_1

1

The economic implications of the pandemic are equally, if not more, dire. According to a Monetary Authority of Singapore (MAS) survey, the Singapore economy is expected to contract by 5.8% in 2020 (CNA 2020). In June 2020, Singapore reported its highest unemployment rate in a decade, with total employment shrinking by 25,600 in the first quarter of 2020 (Phua 2020). This decline in total employment was higher than that during the SARS crisis (24,000) and 2009 Global Financial Crisis (8000).

The impacts of the pandemic has also spilled over into the social sphere, with mental health helplines reporting a surge in number of calls from individuals seeking help and counselling services (Phua and Ang 2020). In all instances, the Covid-19 pandemic has brought forth severe implications for Singapore and posed steep challenges for its policymakers and businesses.

As Prime Minister Lee had mentioned in the above-quoted May Day 2020 message, the Covid-19 pandemic is truly a challenge for Singapore's current generation of policy-makers and citizens. The Prime Minister also alluded in his speech to a set of 'forbearers' whom this current generation is supposedly accountable to. This mention of forbearers is rooted in the understanding that the challenges that Singapore currently faces are not entirely new.

Just 17 years ago, Singapore was affected by the Severe Acute Respiratory Syndrome (SARS) pandemic, which swept through East Asia and infected 238 individuals in Singapore, with 33 of these individuals eventually losing their lives. Similar to the Covid-19 pandemic, the SARS virus had entered Singapore through air travel, with infected persons entering Singapore and subsequently spreading the virus to their close contacts.

More importantly, Singapore's experience with the SARS crisis had yielded valuable policy lessons for its policymakers, with some these lessons culminating in several key policy initiatives and institutional developments that were enacted prior to and during the Covid-19 pandemic. These policy initiatives and institutional developments, what I term policy capacity in this book, have contributed to Singapore's response to the Covid-19 pandemic in many ways.

In this book, I will discuss the policy capacities that were developed in the aftermath of the SARS crisis and which had contributed to the Singapore government's response to the Covid-19 pandemic. These capacities include healthcare infrastructure such as isolation wards, efficient contact tracing processes, and the ability to develop technological tools to assist in the government's Covid-19 response efforts, among many other types of capacities. I will also identify the new policy capacities that were established during and after the Covid-19 pandemic and discuss how these capacities will help prepare Singapore for future pandemics.

At the same time, Singapore's Covid-19 response has also faced several set-backs and limitations. This is especially the case for the large infection clusters that had emerged in the city-state's migrant worker dormitories. As I will discuss in the rest of this book, these shortcomings can mostly be traced to limitations or deficiencies in analytical capacity. These deficiencies had led to the formation of analytical blind-spots, preventing policymakers from accurately assessing the infection risks that resided in Singapore's densely-populated and migrant worker dormitories.

This has in turn given rise to a dual-track outcome in Singapore's Covid-19 response. While the city-state has been successful in minimising Covid-19-related fatalities and curbing the spread of the virus within its citizen population, the formation of large infection clusters in its migrant worker dormitories had given rise to its high infection rates. This raises a further question: how have such high levels of infection occurred in a high-capacity country such as Singapore?

As I will show in the rest of this book, taking a policy capacity approach allows for the deeper understanding of how this dual-track outcome—low fatalities and low community transmission but high rates of infection—had arisen. The story of Singapore's experience with the Covid-19 pandemic is essentially centred on policy capacity, with its success driven by prescient capacity-building efforts and effective mobilisation of these efforts and shortcomings in its early efforts to minimise infection rates attributable to limitations in certain capacities.

Taking a policy capacity approach can therefore provide a clear, objective and systematic understanding of Singapore's Covid-19 response efforts, as well as the areas which policymakers may consider enhancing or strengthening, in order to ensure greater effectiveness in Singapore's future responses to any potential pandemics that may emerge in the horizon.

Beyond Resource Optimisation: Capacity-Building and Robustness

Policy capacity is an emerging analytical framework that is becoming increasingly relevant in public policy scholarly work. I will discuss the emergence of evolution of this theoretical concept in Chapter 2. It suffices for now to say that taking a policy capacity approach allows for a more systematic and policy-oriented approach that focuses on the resources and capacities that policymakers can establish to address future pandemics.

Like all black swan events, pandemics are inherently unpredictable. Despite the best efforts of futurists and scenario planners, it is often impossible to predict the emergence of a global pandemic. However, it is possible to establish ahead of time the institutional and policy capacities that can be mobilised upon the onset of a pandemic. Focusing on policy capacity-building therefore allows policymakers to focus on what they can do, i.e. developing tools and resources, rather than policy goals that cannot be achieved, such as predicting exactly when a pandemic will take place.

It should also be noted that focusing on policy capacity for future pandemics essentially means setting aside excess capacities and resources during ordinary times, with the expectation that these resources and capacities can be quickly mobilised during a pandemic or any other type of crisis. Such an endeavour can be costly and even ideologically problematic, especially with the continued popularity of New Public Management (NPM) practices in governments across the world.

Having emerged in the early 1990s and gained popularity among policy scholars and practitioners through the 2000s, the NPM movement has become the dominant model of public management. At the heart of the NPM movement is an emphasis on cost minimisation and resource optimisation, ostensibly achieved through the contracting out and outsourcing of public services as well as the privatisation of public agencies (Osborne and Gaebler 1993; Dunleavy and Hood 1994; Hood 1995; Pollitt and Bouckaert 2011).

Closely related to the NPM movement is Rational Choice Theory, a public policy theoretical approach that is based on economics and which seeks to model economic and social behaviour on the basis of individual preferences, with these preferences assumed to follow 'rational' and quasi-utilitarian logics of cost minimisation and benefit-maximisation (Ostrom 1991; Stewart 1993, 1993, Neimun and Stambough 1998). From this perspective, government decisions are predicated upon similar logics of cost-minimisation and impact-maximisation.

In any case, idle resources and organisational slack would be anathema to most practitioners and theorists of NPM and Rational Choice Theory. NPM has been particularly popular among governments and policymakers in Southeast Asia (Turner 2002; Samaratunge et al. 2008), with its emphasis on cost reduction and resource optimisation often intersecting neatly with the Asian development state model's focus on economic growth and administrative efficiency (Lee and Haque 2006; Woo 2018). Singapore represents a strong instance of this intersection between NPM and the developmental state model.

The city-state is often held up as the archetypal Asian developmental state, with its adherence to the developmental state model driving its meteoric economic rise (Huff 1995; Perry et al. 1997; Low 2001); it has also over the past few decades introduced many key NPM practices into its Public Service, which has in turn fuelled its reputation for administrative efficiency (Haque 2002; Lee and Haque 2006; Aoki 2015). However, and as I will discuss in the rest of this book, the Covid-19 pandemic has raised important questions over the continued relevance of standard NPM practices in many governments, as well as that of the developmental state model of governance.

For instance, developing and maintaining excess capacity runs counter to NPM's focus on resource optimisation. As I will discuss in Chapters 3 and 4, Singapore had in the aftermath of the SARS crisis expanded the number of isolation wards across its hospitals. It also established the National Centre for Infectious Diseases (NCID), a purpose-built hospital for managing outbreaks of infectious diseases, in 2019. Prior to the Covid-19 pandemic, the NCID was largely involved in research activities, with most of its wards, along with the isolation wards that were established in the other hospitals, relatively under-utilised.

While the presence of such excess healthcare capacity may be seen as a drain on public resources during ordinary times, Singapore's ability to rapidly mobilise these resources during Covid-19 and prevent its healthcare system from being overwhelmed by the large number of Covid-19 infections suggest a need to re-evaluate our existing understandings of resource optimisation and capacity-building. Specifically, there needs to be a certain extent of excess capacity or 'slack' within the healthcare system.

Such 'slack' often takes the form of excess isolation wards, personal protective equipment (PPEs), manpower, and even financial resources, all of which would presumably not be fully utilised during ordinary times but which would play a crucial role in absorbing excess demand for healthcare services during a pandemic. In the case of Singapore, such excess capacity was not limited to its healthcare sector.

Aside from the NCID and the various hospitals' isolation wards that were established post-SARS, Singapore also maintained a 'national stockpile' of food, essential supplies and PPEs. A reserve pool of contact tracing personnel could also be quickly mobilised from the military and the police force, to supplement the contact tracing capabilities of the Ministry of Health. While much of these resources are typically left to sit idle in ordinary times, the emergence of Covid-19 would prompt the rapid mobilisation of these resources. I will discuss this at greater length in Chapter 4.

However, it should be noted that the maintenance of such excess or idle capacity requires large amounts of financial resources, for the maintenance of excess healthcare facilities as well as the building up of stockpiles. Financial resources can also be thought of as another form of excess capacity that can be mobilised to fund governments' policy initiatives during a crisis, as well as purchase more PPEs and essential supplies when excessive demands for these items result in shortages.

In the case of Singapore, such excess financial resources take the form of its large national reserves. Comprising physical assets such as land and buildings and financial assets such as cash, securities and bonds, Singapore's reserves include a substantial amount of 'past reserves' that have been accumulated during previous terms of governments (Ministry of Finance Singapore 2018). Like its excess healthcare capacity and its national stockpile, Singapore's financial reserves represent an intentional effort to set aside excess resources for the future, as opposed to using it for current needs and purposes.

Managed by the Monetary Authority of Singapore, sovereign wealth funds GIC Private Limited and government-owned investment company Temasek Holdings, the total size of Singapore's reserves is a state secret, although analysts have estimated it to be above SG $500 billion (Ng and Jaipragas 2019). The MAS, GIC and Temasek are tasked with reinvesting Singapore's reserves to generate a 'net investment returns contribution' (NIRC) in order to protect these reserves from inflation as well as to generate additional national income.

Taken together, Singapore's national reserves, excess healthcare capacities and national stockpile represent consistent efforts by the government to set aside excess capacities and resources, in anticipation of future needs and crises. This runs counter to traditional NPM thinking, which emphasizes resource optimisation rather than excess capacity or 'slack'. Hence despite its caricatures as a proto-NPM state, Singapore has been in reality building slack into its system, even as it optimises its resources in other areas.

As I will discuss in this book's concluding chapter, it is often not feasible or realistic to understand policy and governance in Singapore through a single theoretical or analytical lens. As the rest of this book will show, taking a capacity approach that focuses on the different resources and capabilities that are mobilised during a policy crisis may be more useful than relying on broad normative theoretical frameworks such as the developmental state model or NPM.

Singapore's efforts to maintain excess capacity and slack also speak to another analytical concept that has been gaining interest in the study of crisis management: robustness. Robustness has been described as "ability to withstand or survive external shocks, to be stable in spite of uncertainty" (Bankes 2010, p. 2), or the "ability of a system to withstand perturbations in structure without change in function" (Jen 2003, p. 14).

Robustness can also exist in public agencies and organisations, with organisational robustness described as the "capacity of an organization to retain its fundamental pattern at core characteristics under changing conditions" (van Oss and van 't Hek 2011, p. 34). In my earlier work, I had defined robustness in a policy system as:

> a property of the institutional arrangements through which a system can adapt or can regain stability after having encountered periods of uncertainty and/or transformation. Unlike resilience, the stability that a robust system regains after recovering from shock and uncertainty may not resemble its pre-shock state. This nature of robustness therefore allows it to be considered a characteristic that is manipulable by agents and, thus, is subject to policy design and redesign. (Capano and Woo 2017).

In sum, a robust policy system is one that is able to retain functionality amidst shocks and crisis, sometimes by withstanding shocks but more often by adapting to these shocks and hence shifting to a 'new normal'. Whereas resilience tends to focus on 'rebounding' from a crisis, robustness emphasizes operating or functioning through crises. As I have also noted in my other writings, this focus on rebounding can result in a certain extent of rigidity in a policy system, since a system that has rebounded to its pre-crisis state would likely have recreated the very sources of its vulnerability (Capano and Woo 2017, 2018).

These insights pose significant implications for the study of crises and pandemics. While resilience is typically emphasized in studies of crisis management, with the aim of removing the source of instability and returning to pre-crisis conditions, robustness is more aligned with the findings and expectations of policy capacity, since capacity-building involves establishing the resources and capabilities for dealing with crisis or maintaining policy functionality during a crisis. Robustness therefore represents a key guiding principle underlying this book's focus on capacity-building for pandemic response.

Similar to capacity-building, building up robustness in a policy system may at times require a shift away from resource optimisation. For instance, the policy scientist John Dryzek has called for the replacement of optimisation as the guiding principle for policy design with robustness, since a "a robust policy alternative is one expected to perform tolerably well across the whole range of scenarios" (Dryzek 1983, pp. 360–361). This suggests the need for some level of slack, with robust policy alternatives capable of withstanding a certain range of variation or shock.

As I will consistently argue in the rest of this book, robust systems and robust responses to pandemics and crisis require the maintenance of excess capacity. This allows policy systems to mobilise excess resources and retain systemic functionality during a shock or crisis. Before proceeding to discuss capacity and robustness in Singapore's pandemic and crisis response measures, I will first provide a brief overview of Singapore's policy and governance system.

SINGAPORE: A BRIEF PRIMER

The contours of Singapore's geographical, demographic and socio-economic realities are familiar to many. Located on the tip of the Malaysian peninsular along the Strait of Malacca, Singapore straddles important trade routes between the East and West. It is this strategic location that had led the British to establish a Crown colony in Singapore. As I will discuss below, this period of British colonial rule would deeply influence Singapore's political system.

In any case, Singapore's experience with British colonial rule would be interrupted by Japanese invasion and occupation during the Second World War in 1945, with the post-war return of British rule cut short by Singapore's merger with Malaysia in 1963. This merger would also prove short-lived, with deep political and economic differences between the governments of Singapore and Malaysia giving rise to a separation that would result in Singapore becoming an independent and sovereign state on 9 August 1965.

Singapore has since its independence transformed itself into a global city with a thriving economy. As of 2019, Singapore's Gross Domestic Product (GDP) per capita stands at US$65,233 (World Bank 2020). As a point of comparison, Singapore's GDP per capita is slightly higher than that of the United States, which is currently US$65,281. Singapore's economy is also ranked the most competitive in the world (IMD 2020).

Singapore's economic success is driven by an economic policy stance that has emphasized economic openness. This began at independence, when the government deliberately encouraged multinational corporations to set up their offices and operations in Singapore. This led to an extended period of export-led growth, which drove the industrialisation of Singapore's economy. However, the emergence of regional manufacturing powerhouses such as China would prompt the Singapore government develop its services sector as a second 'engine' for its economy.

This search for a second 'engine' led first to the establishment of Singapore's financial services sector in the early 1970s, with financial services seen as an 'exportable service' that could contribute to Singapore's economic development (Woo 2016). Other sectors that were subsequently developed included biotechnology and pharmaceuticals, tourism, and more recently, technology. Driven by its Smart Nation initiative, Singapore's technology sector has brought forth wide-ranging implications for its other sectors and industries.

At the same time, the constraints that Singapore has always faced remain. This includes a lack of natural resources[1], limited physical territory and a small population. Singapore's currently has a population of close to 5.7 million while its total land area is approximately 724 km^2. As I will discuss in the following chapters, Singapore's economic openness, especially its reliance on international trade and tourism, has also made it vulnerable to the spread of infectious diseases.

The rapid development of Singapore's economy despite these physical constraints has often been attributed to its model of policy and governance, which is known for its transparency and administrative efficiency.

---

[1] While Singapore has achieved a significant extent of self-reliance in its water needs through desalination and treating reclaimed wastewater, it continues to purchase water from Malaysia.

I will now turn my attention to Singapore's political system and policy processes.

At the heart of Singaporean governance is its Westminster parliamentary system and the ruling People's Action Party (PAP), which has won every election since independence. Often seen as a legacy of its British colonial history, Singapore's parliamentary system retains its majoritarian and first-past-the-post characteristics, with Members of Parliament (MPs) elected into parliament by through General Elections that must be held once every five years.

Like all parliamentary systems, the political party that wins the most seats gets to form the government, with the Prime Minister and his cabinet drawn from the ruling party's elected MPs. Parliament therefore forms Singapore's Legislature, with bills and laws debated and passed in the House, while the Prime Minister and his cabinet make up the Executive. Singapore's judiciary is made up of its courts. It should be noted that several modifications have been made to Singapore's parliamentary system, with the aim of introducing greater diversity and representativeness.

These include the introduction of a popularly-elected President whose role it is to safeguard Singapore's national reserves, a Group Representative Constituency system that requires voters to choose between competing teams of political candidates (with the entire team voted in at the same time), non-constituency members of parliament (NCMPs) who are drawn from the 'best-losing' opposition candidates but enjoy equal voting rights with elected MPs, and nominated members of parliament (NMPs) who are appointed by the President to represent specific sectors of society that may not be sufficiently represented by political parties, such as the Arts or the disabled (Singh 2012; Tan 2013).

Once they have been appointed to the Cabinet, Ministers are in charge of specific ministries and their statutory boards. For instance, the Minister of Health is tasked with leading the Ministry of Health and its various statutory boards, such as the Health Promotion Board and Health Sciences Authorities, among others. Junior ministers are also often appointed to each ministry. These are known as Ministers of State or Senior Ministers of State. The public servants who form the various ministries therefore report to the Minister, with the most senior of these being the Permanent Secretary. Statutory boards are typically led by Chief Executive who report to the Permanent Secretary.

Singapore's Public Service is known for its administrative efficiency and transparency, with the latter driven by the PAP's zero tolerance approach to corruption (Quah 1995, 2001, 2013; Jones 1999; Haque 2009). Policymaking in Singapore is also highly performance-driven. This is due in part to the city-state's adherence to the Asian developmental state model of governance that emphasizes performance legitimacy (Low 2001; Liow 2011; Woo 2018) and in part to the government's conscious efforts to introduce New Public Management (NPM) practices to its public service (Haque 2002; Lee and Haque 2006; Aoki 2015).

NPM has since become a dominant driver of Singapore's public service and its policy processes. This is especially evident in the privatization and corporatization of several public agencies and statutory boards, giving rise to 'government-linked companies' (GLCs) that serve to provide some form of public service in 'strategic sectors' such as Singapore Technology Engineering (ST Engineering), Singapore International Airlines (SIA) and Singapore Telecommunications (SingTel), among others.

Aside from privatization, the government also adopted private sector management practices in its public service. This includes performance-based management and budgeting, decentralisation of more competitive recruitment and promotion criteria, efforts to encourage innovation in the public sector, and a greater focus on customer service. These practices have in turn further contributed to greater efficiency in the public service.

HEALTHCARE SYSTEM

According to the Economist Intelligence Unit's Healthcare Outcomes Index, Singapore's healthcare system is ranked 2nd out of 166 in the world, with Japan taking the top spot (The Economist Intelligence Unit 2014). Singapore's healthcare system is also ranked the second most efficient in the world on the Bloomberg Heath Care Efficiency Index while a Philips survey of 16 countries finds that Singapore's healthcare system offers the best value and is the most future-proof (*Singapore Business Review* 2018; Wong 2018).

Singapore's healthcare system has also driven its emergence as a leading global healthcare hub, with medical tourism contributing to Singapore's overall economic development and competitiveness (Pocock and Phua 2011; Ganguli and Ebrahim 2017). In the rest of this section, I will provide a brief overview of Singapore's healthcare system and the fundamental tenets of its healthcare policy.

Singapore's healthcare system is governed and regulated by the Ministry of Health (MOH) and its statutory boards. These statutory boards include the Health Promotion Board, Health Sciences Authority Singapore Nursing Board, Singapore Dental Council, Singapore Medical Council, Singapore Pharmacy Council, and the Traditional Chinese Medicine Practitioners Board. Statutory boards are semi-autonomous public agencies that operate under the purview of specific ministries (Lee 1975; Woo 2014).

Under this system, all healthcare facilities, such as hospitals, medical centres, community health centres and polyclinics, nursing homes, primary care clinics, dental clinics and clinical laboratories are required to be licensed under the Private Hospitals & Medical Clinics (PHMC) Act/Regulations. The PHMC Act/Regulations also regulate the quality and standard of medical services provided by these facilities.

Taken together, Singapore's medical facilities form a broad tapestry of healthcare providers, with each type of provider providing different level or form healthcare service. At the centre of these facilities are Singapore's hospitals. Table 1.1 lists the number of hospitals in Singapore.

Acute hospitals include General Hospitals that provide multi-disciplinary acute inpatient and specialist outpatient service, a women's and children's hospital (which was restructured from the KKH), a multi-disciplinary hospital and a tertiary hospital that also serves as a major research centre. These are listed in Table 1.2.

The government has more recently revealed that a 12th public hospital, serving both acute care and community roles, will be established in Eastern Singapore by 2030 while another new public hospital is expected to be completed in Northern Singapore in 2022 (Khalik 2020). Such efforts to geographically distribute hospitals across Singapore are not new. The siting and development of public hospitals in Singapore is strongly

Table 1.1 Singapore's hospitals

		Acute hospitals	Psychiatric hospitals	Community hospitals
	Public	10	1	5
	Private	8	0	0
	Not-for-profit	1	0	4

Adapted from Ministry of Health (2020), "Health Facilities" (Ministry of Health 2020a)

Table 1.2   Acute hospitals

Hospital	Type	Healthcare cluster
Singapore General Hospital	General	SingHealth
Changi General Hospital	General	SingHealth
Sengkang General Hospital	General	SingHealth
Khoo Teck Puat Hospital	General	National Healthcare Group
Ng Teng Fong General Hospital	General	National University Health System
Alexandra Hospital	General	National University Health System
Tan Tock Seng Hospital	Multi-Disciplinary	National Healthcare Group
National University Hospital	Tertiary and Research	National University Health System
Kadang Kerbau Women's and Children's Hospital	Women's and Children's	SingHealth

Source Ministry of Health Singapore https://www.moh.gov.sg/home/our-healthcare-system

linked to its urban policies, with each hospital expected to cater to the healthcare needs of a specific district or neighbourhood.

Aside from geographical distribution, Singapore's public hospitals are also organised and managed within several healthcare 'clusters'. As Table 1.2 shows, Singapore's public hospitals belong to several healthcare clusters, namely SingHealth, the National Healthcare Group, and the National University Health System. The presence of these three different health clusters reflect a significant extent of decentralisation and diversification in Singapore's delivery of its healthcare services.

This began with the National Healthcare Plan, which was unveiled in 1983 to introduce significant reforms to Singapore's healthcare system. While the Plan and other subsequent early efforts gave rise to six healthcare clusters that decentralised the management of healthcare facilities and delivery of public services, a public healthcare reorganisation that was carried out in 2017 resulted in a merger of several clusters to form the three major clusters of SingHealth, National Healthcare Group and the National University Health System (Poon 2017).

Aside from public hospitals, each public healthcare cluster also oversees a range of national specialty centres and polyclinics. Polyclinics are public 'one-stop' health centres that provide subsidised primary health-care services, alongside approximately private 1700 General Practitioner (GP) clinics that provide the bulk of Singapore's primary healthcare services (Ministry of Health 2020b). The three public healthcare clusters and their constituent healthcare institutions are listed in Table 1.3.

At the organisational level, the National Healthcare Plan also gave rise to extensive restructuring and corporatisation of Singapore's public hospitals, in the process granting them greater autonomy in their day-to-day operations and management as well as introducing a significant extent of competition in the public healthcare system (Haseltine 2013, p. 10). Beginning with the National University hospital in 1985 and the Singapore General hospital in 1989, most of the public hospitals were corporatized by the end of the 1990s.

The National Healthcare Plan also laid the foundations for universal health coverage. This began with the introduction of the Medisave plan, which is essentially a compulsory savings account under the CPF system that can be drawn on to pay for major medical costs incurred by the account holder and his/her immediate family members. Under this system, a certain portion of the CPF member's monthly contributions are allocated to the Medisave account, to be used exclusively for medical expenses. The Medisave allocations can range from 8% for members aged 35 and below to 10.5% for members aged 50 and above(Central Provident Fund Board 2020).

While the MediSave system has since been expanded to allow accoun-tholders to draw on MediSave funds to pay for medical expenses incurred in approved private hospitals as well as pay for all categories of hospital room charges, it was increasingly clear that MediSave alone was not enough to cover high-cost medical expenditures (Phua 2018, p. 37). In response, MediShield was introduced in 1990 as a form of limited health insurance that covers either very long hospital stays or certain costly outpatient treatments, with MediShield premiums automatically deducted from MediSave.

Supplementary plans such as MediShield Plus and Private Medical Insurance Schemes were also introduced in 1994 to allow for different levels of coverage and claims thresholds while private insurance firms began offering Integrated Shield Plans that could be purchased to add on private supplementary insurance to the basic public plans. These Inte-grated Shield Plans often provide much greater coverage than the basic

Table 1.3 Public healthcare clusters

	SingHealth	National Healthcare Group	National University Health System
Hospitals	• Singapore General Hospital • KK Women's and Children's Hospital • Changi General Hospital • Sengkang General Hospital • Bright Vision Hospital • Outram Community Hospital • Sengkang Community Hospital	• Tan Tock Seng Hospital • Khoo Teck Puat Hospital • Institute of Mental Health • Yishun Community Hospital	• National University Hospital • Ng Teng Fong General Hospital • Jurong Community Hospital • Alexandra Hospital
Specialist centres	• Singapore National Eye Centre • National Cancer Centre Singapore • National Heart Centre Singapore • National Dental Centre Singapore • National Neuroscience Institute	• National Skin Centre	• National University Cancer Institute, Singapore • National University Heart Centre, Singapore • National University Centre for Oral Health, Singapore
Polyclinics	• Bedok • Bukit Merah • Marine Parade • Outram • Pasir Ris • Punggol • Sengkang • Tampines	• Ang Mo Kio • Hougang • Woodlands • Geylang • Toa Payoh • Yishun	• Bukit Batok • Bukit Panjang • Clementi • Choa Chu Kang • Jurong • Pioneer • Queenstown

Source Ministry of Health Singapore https://www.moh.gov.sg/home/our-healthcare-system

public plans, with higher-tiered plans allowing for medical claims on an 'as-charged' basis, rather than imposing a ceiling on allowable claims.

The MediShield system would be significantly upgraded with the introduction of MediShield Life in 2015, which functions as a lifetime universal health insurance scheme that helps pay for large hospital bills and selected costly outpatient treatments such as dialysis or chemotherapy for cancer (Ministry of Health 2019). Lastly, Medifund was introduced in 1993 as a government endowment fund to help those who are unable to afford subsidised medical charges, even after MediSave and MediShield Life. As a supplement, ElderShield was also introduced in 2002 to provide long-term disability insurance for Singapore's growing elderly population.

MediSave, MediShield Life and MediFund form the '3 Ms' of Singapore's healthcare financing system, which emphasizes personal responsibility over state expenditures by ensuring a largely self-funded healthcare financing system (Phua 2018, pp. 35–36). Hence while the 3Ms introduced universal health coverage in Singapore, this coverage is largely funded by citizens' MediSave funds rather than direct state spending.

Aside from providing for the healthcare needs of its citizens, Singapore's healthcare system also forms the core of Singapore's emergence as a leading global healthcare hub (Pocock and Phua 2011; Ganguli and Ebrahim 2017). Indeed, the healthcare reforms that have been discussed above are seen to have contributed immensely to Singapore's success as a healthcare hub, with the efficiency and quality of its hospitals and specialist centres serving to attract 'medical tourists' from across the world, many of whom come to Singapore exclusively to seek medical treatment (Leng 2010; Koh and Cheah 2015).

At the same time, Singapore's position as a global travel node and healthcare hub has also made it vulnerable to the spread of infectious diseases. While the first cases of SARS and Covid-19 came from individuals who had travelled from Hong Kong and Wuhan respectively, two imported cases of Covid-19 had arrived in Singapore to seek treatment, after having reported coronavirus symptoms in Indonesia (Aravindan and Geddie 2020).

Nonetheless, Singapore's highly developed healthcare system has allowed it to weather the SARS and Covid-19 pandemics. As I will discuss in the following chapters, Singapore's healthcare policy capacities, developed over the course of its healthcare reform and augmented with its experience with SARS, has allowed the city-state to respond quickly to the Covid-19 crisis. This reflects a high level of robustness in Singapore's healthcare system. Such robustness stems from the Singapore government's efforts at policy capacity-building.

Outline of the Book

This chapter has provided a broad overview of Singapore's approach to policy and governance and situated it within broader policy theoretical constructs such as robustness and capacity. It has also laid out the contours of Singapore's healthcare system. As I will discuss in the following chapters, the robustness of Singapore's policy processes and its healthcare system, driven by the government's capacity-building efforts, has allowed it to respond quickly to the Covid-19 pandemic. In the following chapters, I will discuss policy capacity and Singapore's pandemic response efforts at greater length.

This will begin with a deep and systematic review of the policy capacity literature in Chapter 2. As a theoretical framework, policy capacity is fairly new. By drawing on this emerging policy framework, this chapter will engage with an emerging set of cutting edge research on policy capacity and design. This is followed by a brief discussion of Singapore's response to the SARS pandemic in Chapter 3, with a specific focus on the institutional and policy capacities that were established after the 2003 SARS crisis. By delineating and categorising these capacities, this chapter provides a broad overview of Singapore's pandemic response processes and procedures, much of which were established in response to the SARS crisis.

This will form an important backdrop for Chapter 4's discussions on Singapore's response to the Covid-19 pandemic. In this chapter, I will discuss Singapore's response to the Covid-19 pandemic, focusing in particular on how it has mobilised and adapted its policy capacities to deal with the pandemic. I will also discuss the new capacities that were established this period. In focusing on how policy capacities were drawn upon or created in its Covid-19 response, this chapter will provide readers with an understanding of the various policy capacities that are necessary for responding to pandemics and other healthcare crises.

In Chapter 5, I will provide readers with a brief summary of the key arguments and findings that have been presented in the previous chapters. This will allow me to present a broad policy capacity framework that will be useful for policymakers and practitioners who may be interested in building up the necessary capacities for dealing with future pandemics. I will also discuss potential areas for future research and theorising.

This book is by no means the final word on Singapore's pandemic response efforts. Rather, it aims to provide a useful first step for further research on the subject, much of which will no doubt continue to be informed by further developments in the ongoing Covid-19 crisis and Singapore's continued efforts to manage the impacts of this pandemic.

REFERENCES

Aoki, N. (2015). Institutionalization of New Public Management: The Case of Singapore's Education System. *Public Management Review, 17*(2), 165–186.
Aravindan, A., & Geddie, J. (2020, March 10). *Singapore Charges Visitors for Coronavirus Treatment After Imported Indonesian Cases*. Reuters.
Bankes, S. (2010). *Robustness, Adaptivity, and Resiliency Analysis*.
Capano, G., & Woo, J. J. (2017). Resilience and Robustness in Policy Design: A Critical Appraisal. *Policy Sciences, 50*, 1–28.
Capano, G., & Woo, J. J. (2018). Designing Policy Robustness: Outputs and Processes. *Policy and Society, 37*(4), 422–440.
Central Provident Fund Board. (2020). *MediSave* [online]. Available from: https://www.cpf.gov.sg/Members/Schemes/schemes/healthcare/med isave. Accessed 19 April 2020.
CNA. (2020). *Singapore GDP Forecast to Contract by 5.8% in 2020: MAS Survey* [online]. CNA. Available from: https://www.channelnewsasia.com/ news/business/economy-gdp-mas-forecast-survey-q2-12835070. Accessed 22 June 2020.
Dryzek, J. S. (1983). Don't Toss Coins in Garbage Cans: A Prologue to Policy Design. *Journal of Public Policy, 3*(4), 345–367.
Dunleavy, P., & Hood, C. (1994). From Old Public Administration to New Public Management. *Public Money & Management, 14*(3), 9–16.
Ganguli, S., & Ebrahim, A. H. (2017). A Qualitative Analysis of Singapore's Medical Tourism Competitiveness. *Tourism Management Perspectives, 21*, 74–84.
Haque, M. S. (2002). Structures of New Public Management in Malaysia and Singapore: Alternative Views. *The Journal of Comparative Asian Development, 1*(1), 71–86.
Haque, M. S. (2009). Public Administration and Public Governance in Singapore. In P. S. Kim (Ed.), *Public Administration and Public Governance in ASEAN and Korea* (pp. 246–271). Seoul: Daeyong Moonhwasa Publishing Company.
Haseltine, W. A. (2013). *Affordable Excellence: The Singapore Healthcare Story: How to Create and Manage Sustainable Healthcare Systems*. Washington, DC: Brookings Institution Press.
Hood, C. (1995). The "New Public Management" in the 1980s: Variations on a Theme. *Accounting, Organizations and Society, 20*(2–3), 93–109.

Huff, W. G. (1995). The Developmental State, Government, and Singapore's Economic Development Since 1960. *World Development, 23*(8), 1421–1438.

IMD. (2020). *World Competitiveness Ranking.* Lausanne, Switzerland: IMD.

Jen, E. (2003). Stable or Robust? What's the Difference? *Complexity, 8*(3), 12–18.

Jones, D. S. (1999). Public Administration in Singapore: Continuity and Reform. In H. K. Wong & H. S. Chan (Eds.), *Handbook of Comparative Public Administration in the Asia-Pacific Basin* (pp. 1–22). New York: CRC Press.

Khalik, S. (2020). New Hospital in the East; Alexandra to Be Expanded [online]. *The Straits Times.* Available from: https://www.straitstimes.com/singapore/new-hospital-in-the-east-alexandra-to-be-expanded. Accessed 20 April 2020.

Koh, A., & Cheah, J. (2015). No Hospital Is an Island—Emerging New Roles of the Acute General Hospital in the Singapore Healthcare Ecosystem. *Future Hospital Journal, 2*(2), 121–124.

Lee, B. H. (1975). *Statutory Boards in Singapore.* Singapore: Department of Political Science, University of Singapore.

Lee, E. W. Y., & Haque, M. S. (2006). The New Public Management Reform and Governance in Asian NICs: A Comparison of Hong Kong and Singapore. *Governance, 19*(4), 605–626.

Leng, C. H. (2010). Medical Tourism and the State in Malaysia and Singapore. *Global Social Policy, 10*(3), 336–357.

Liow, E. D. (2011). The Neoliberal-Developmental State: Singapore as Case Study. *Critical Sociology.* https://doi.org/10.1177/0896920511419900.

Low, L. (2001). The Singapore Developmental State in the New Economy and Polity. *The Pacific Review, 14*(3), 411–441.

Ministry of Finance Singapore. (2018). *Our Nation's Reserves* [online]. Available from: https://www.mof.gov.sg/policies/our-nation's-reserves/Section-I-What-comprises-the-reserves-and-who-manages-them. Accessed 25 June 2020.

Ministry of Health. (2019). *MediShield Life* [online]. Ministry of Health Singapore. Available from: https://www.moh.gov.sg/cost-financing/healthcare-schemes-subsidies/medishield-life. Accessed 14 September 2016.

Ministry of Health. (2020a). *MOH | Healthcare Services and Facilities* [online]. Ministry of Health Singapore. Available from: https://www.moh.gov.sg/home/our-healthcare-system/healthcare-services-and-facilities. Accessed 18 April 2020.

Ministry of Health. (2020b). *MOH | Primary Healthcare Services* [online]. Ministry of Health Singapore. Available from: https://www.moh.gov.sg/home/our-healthcare-system/healthcare-services-and-facilities/primary-healthcare-services. Accessed 20 April 2020.

Neimun, M., & Stambough, S. J. (1998). Rational Choice Theory and the Evaluation of Public Policy. *Policy Studies Journal, 26*(3), 449–465.

Ng, J. Y., & Jaipragas, B. (2019). Singapore's Giant Reserves: A Taxing Question for Heng Swee Keat [online]. *South China Morning Post*. Available from: https://www.scmp.com/week-asia/politics/article/2186409/sin gapores-giant-reserves-taxing-question-its-next-prime-minister. Accessed 12 May 2020.

Osborne, D., & Gaebler, T. (1993). *Reinventing Government: How the Entrepreneurial Spirit Is Transforming the Public Sector*. New York, NY: Plume.

Ostrom, E. (1991). Rational Choice Theory and Institutional Analysis: Toward Complementarity. *American Political Science Review, 85*(1), 237–243.

Perry, M., Kong, L., & Yeoh, B. (1997). *Singapore: A Developmental City State*. Chichester: Wiley.

Phua, K. H. (2018). *Healthcare*. Singapore: Straits Times Press.

Phua, R. (2020). *Singapore's Jobless Rate Highest in 10 Years, Total Employment Registers Record Decline in Q1* [online]. CNA. Available from: https://www. channelnewsasia.com/news/singapore/unemployment-jobless-highest-10-years-retrenchments-mom-12835166. Accessed 22 June 2020.

Phua, R., & Ang, H. M. (2020). *COVID-19: Worries About Pandemic See More Calls to Mental Health Helplines* [online]. CNA. Available from: https:// www.channelnewsasia.com/news/singapore/covid-19-fear-toll-mental-hea lth-hotline-anxiety-singapore-12631710. Accessed 22 June 2020.

Pocock, N. S., & Phua, K. H. (2011). Medical Tourism and Policy Implications for Health Systems: A Conceptual Framework from a Comparative Study of Thailand, Singapore and Malaysia. *Globalization and Health, 7*(1), 12.

Pollitt, C., & Bouckaert, G. (2011). *Public Management Reform: A Comparative Analysis—New Public Management, Governance, and the Neo-Weberian State* (3rd ed.). Oxford and New York: Oxford University Press.

Poon, C. H. (2017). Public Healthcare Sector to be Reorganised into 3 Integrated Clusters, New Polyclinic Group to Be Formed [online]. *The Straits Times*. Available from: https://www.straitstimes.com/singapore/health/public-healthcare-sector-to-be-reorganised-into-3-integrated-cluste rs-new. Accessed 7 July 2020.

Quah, J. S. T. (1995). Sustaining Quality in the Singapore Civil Service. *Public Administration and Development, 15*(3), 335–343.

Quah, J. S. T. (2001). Combating Corruption in Singapore: What Can Be Learned? *Journal of Contingencies and Crisis Management, 9*(1), 29–35.

Quah, J. S. T. (2013). Ensuring Good Governance in Singapore: Is This Experience Transferable to Other Asian Countries? *International Journal of Public Sector Management, 26*(5), 401–420.

Samaratunge, R., Alam, Q., & Teicher, J. (2008). The New Public Management Reforms in Asia: A Comparison of South and Southeast Asian Countries. *International Review of Administrative Sciences, 74*(1), 25–46.

Singapore Business Review. (2018). Singapore Dethroned by Hong Kong as World's Most Efficient Healthcare System: Bloomberg [online]. *Singapore Business Review*. Available from: https://sbr.com.sg/healthcare/news/sin gapore-dethroned-hong-kong-worlds-most-efficient-healthcare-system-blo omberg. Accessed 18 April 2020.

Singh, B. (2012). *Politics and Governance in Singapore: An Introduction* (2nd ed.). Singapore: McGraw-Hill Education (Asia).

Stewart, J. (1993). Rational Choice Theory, Public Policy and the Liberal State. *Policy Sciences, 26*(4), 317–330.

Tan, K. P. (2013). The Singapore Parliament: Representation, Effectiveness, and Control. In Y. Zheng, L. F. Lye, & W. Hofmeister (Eds.), *Parliaments in Asia: Institutional Building and Political Development* (pp. 27–46). Oxford, UK: Routledge.

The Economist Intelligence Unit. (2014). *Healthcare Outcomes Index 2014* [online]. Available from: https://www.eiu.com/public/topical_report.aspx?campaignid=Healthoutcome2014. Accessed 18 April 2020.

Turner, M. (2002). Choosing Items from the Menu: New Public Management in Southeast Asia. *International Journal of Public Administration, 25*(12), 1493–1512.

van Oss, L., & van 't Hek, J. (2011). *Why Organizational Change Fails: Robustness, Tenacity, and Change in Organizations* (1st ed.). New York: Routledge.

Wong, P. T. (2018). *S'pore's Healthcare System Best in Value and Satisfaction, but Falls Behind in Providing Access: Study—TODAY online* [online]. Available from: https://www.todayonline.com/singapore/spores-healthcare-system-best-value-and-satisfaction-falls-behind-providing-access-study. Accessed 18 April 2020.

Woo, J. J. (2014). Singapore's Policy Style: Statutory Boards as Policymaking Units. *Journal of Asian Public Policy, 8*(2), 120–133.

Woo, J. J. (2016). *Singapore as an International Financial Centre: History, Politics and Policy.* London: Palgrave Macmillan.

Woo, J. J. (2018). *The Evolution of the Asian Developmental State: Hong Kong and Singapore.* London: Routledge.

World Bank. (2020). *GDP per capita (current US$)—Singapore | Data* [online]. Available from: https://data.worldbank.org/indicator/NY.GDP.PCAP.CD?locations=SG. Accessed 7 July 2020.

CHAPTER 2

Policy Capacity

Abstract In this chapter, I will provide readers with a comprehensive understanding of policy capacity. This includes a broad overview of the existing theoretical and empirical literature on policy capacity. As a theoretical framework, policy capacity is fairly new. By drawing on this emerging policy framework, this chapter will engage with an emerging set of cutting edge research on policy capacity and design.

Keywords Policy capacity · Policy design · Robustness · Resilience

Policy capacity is a relatively new framework for policy analysis, although it has of late gained much attention and interest among policy scholars and practitioners. Much of this has to do with the 2009 Global Financial Crisis, which had prompted policy scholars to pay closer attention to the government competencies and capabilities that are required to prevent, or mitigate the impacts of, such crises (Howlett and Lejano 2013; Howlett et al. 2015). However, the idea of capacity in a state's policy processes is not entirely new.

Scholars of international relations and security studies have long focused on the state's monopoly over the exercise of legitimate force within its territorial boundaries as the key indicator of state capacity (Weber 1919). Much of these studies of 'state strength' have therefore

© The Author(s), under exclusive license to Springer Nature   23
Singapore Pte Ltd. 2021
J. J. Woo, *Capacity-building and Pandemics*,
https://doi.org/10.1007/978-981-15-9453-3_2

tended to focus on the state's ability to either ensure domestic stability or define its territories from foreign invasion (Sørensen 1993; Seabrooke 2002; Volgy and Bailin 2003; Taylor and Botea 2008). Military and policing capabilities therefore take centre stage in these studies of capacity (Fearon and Laitin 2003), particularly in realist perspectives that place a strong premium on 'state strength' as a means of securing domestic policy objectives (Waltz 1954; Krasner 1976; Holsti and Holsti 1996; Volgy and Bailin 2003). Conversely, states that lack such strength or capacity are often described by international relations scholars as 'failed states' that lack of the financial, organisational and political capacities needed for maintaining governmental functionality (Rotberg 2002; Hameiri 2007; Besley and Persson 2008).

These insights are highly relevant for the case of Singapore, with its realist approach to international relations driving the creation of its formidable military force and informing its ongoing efforts to emphasize the rule of law in domestic and regional affairs (Leifer 2000; Ganesan 2005; Guo and Woo 2016). These capabilities have no doubt proven useful during the Covid-19 pandemic, especially in terms of the severe penalties for flouting safety distancing rules and the mobilisation of military personnel and resources for contact tracing, distribution of masks to the general public, and providing medical care to migrant worker dormitories (Lim 2020; Mahmud 2020; Tee 2020).

More importantly, Singapore's realist approach to managing crises also means that external crises (actual or anticipated) tend to give rise to extensive capacity-building efforts, often in anticipation of future crises (Leifer 2000). The 'siege mentality' that has often been associated with Singapore's realist approach to international relations has also spurred its efforts at capacity-building, with its formidable military, national stockpile and sizeable national reserves being cases in point (Leifer 2000; Ganesan 2005).

However, such military-focused and legalistic understandings of state strength can also be analytically-limiting. Indeed, capacity-building efforts often also include non-realist tools such as alliance-building or participation in multilateral organisations. In many instances, such liberal approaches to international relations, while not necessarily contributing to the building up of state military capacities, contribute to another equally important facet of state capacity: economic power.

Fundamental to any country's survival is its ability to ensure economic growth and employment. It is therefore hardly surprising that many early efforts to understand state capacity were focused on the state's ability to ensure economic growth and employment for its citizens (Skocpol and Finegold 1982; Evans 1995; Weiss and Hobson 1995; World Bank 1997). Such understandings of capacity tend to associate capacity with economic performance, with quantifiable measures such as GDP growth rates, unemployment rates and inflation levels frequently used by policy analysts and citizens alike as convenient proxies of state capacity.

This focus on economic growth and performance is particularly pronounced in the developmental state literature, which emphasizes economic performance as both barometer of state strength and source of political legitimacy (Johnson 1982; Evans 1989; Douglass 1994; Leftwich 1995; Woo-Cumings 1999). Indeed, East Asian developmental states such as Japan, South Korea, Singapore, Taiwan and China have often been held up as paragons of high-capacity states (Chu 2016; Hellmann 2018; Woo 2018), with their rapid rise in the regional and global economy seen as a result of their respective governments' effective economic policymaking.

According to the developmental state scholar Peter Evans, the ongoing efforts of these developmental states to expand or enhance their economic policy capacities also makes them 'capacity-enhancing states' (Evans 2014). Such efforts at constant capacity-enhancement is no doubt driven by the intense economic competition that has arisen among East Asian states, all of which had taken on export-led strategies to drive economic growth in the formative years of their development. This meant constant efforts by policymakers to enhance domestic infrastructural conditions and productive capacities in a bid to enhance their respective economies' competitiveness vis-à-vis other East Asian developmental states.

Aside from the success of its economic reform policies, the success of the developmental state model also depends on the internal coherency of its public agencies and bureaucracy, or what is known in the Weberian tradition as 'bureaucratic rationality', with a highly disciplined civil service that is capable of close inter-agency cooperation seen as a key determinant of success (Chibber 2002). There is therefore an administrative or operational aspect of capacity in the developmental state, with state capacity dependent on the administrative efficiency and policy efficacy of its pilot agencies.

Yet at the same time, an understanding of state capacity that is predicated solely on economic performance can have its limits. For instance, the onset of globalization and the emergence of powerful private actors as well as the proliferation of neoliberal economic ideologies are seen to have resulted in the decline of state capacity among major developmental states (Strange 1996; Cutler et al. 1999; Haufler 2001; Cutler 2003). However, even amidst such extensive globalisation, developmental states such as South Korean, China, Singapore and Hong Kong have retained their economic strength and even managed to build up their 'soft power' (Nye 2005; Wang 2008; Lee 2009; Chong 2010; Bräutigam and Xiaoyang 2012).

A more plausible view would be that globalization has not given rise to a decline in state capacity insomuch as it has prompted states to recalibrate the forms of capacity that they are able to draw on (Weiss 1998, 2000). Indeed, the challenges that have emerged with globalisation have given rise to greater imperatives for state action, particularly among developmental states that remain intent on determining economic growth in an increasingly globalised and hyper-competitive economy (Ramesh 1995; Perraton 2005).

There is therefore a need for a broader understanding of capacity that takes into account the various economic and non-economic aspects of policy and governance as well as the different modalities through which state power and authority are exercised. To this end, a growing body of research has sought to provide a broader understanding of 'policy capacity' that cuts across specific policy domains to encompass the broader policy process.

POLICY CAPACITY

Drawn from the policy sciences discipline, these more contemporaneous understandings of capacity initially focused on the various aspects or stages of the policy process, such as decision-making and the ability to assess multiple policy alternatives (Bakvis 2000; Painter and Pierre 2005), horizon scanning and the setting of strategic directions (Howlett and Lindquist 2004) or the appropriate application of knowledge in policy-making (Parsons 2004). Others sought to take a more organisational and administrative perspective, where capacity is often thought of in terms of public agencies' ability to coordinate and implement public service delivery (World Bank 2012, 2014; Holt and Manning 2014).

A growing recognition of a need to think about policy capacity in terms of both outcomes (policy effectiveness) and capabilities (resources and institutions) (Mukherjee and Bali 2019) would give rise to a growing body of work that sought to identify and categorise the different types of capacities that governments have at their disposal. This shift in focus on measuring policy outcomes to identifying capabilities naturally prompted scholars to build up typologies of capacities. The policy capacities that have thus far been identified in the existing literature include political, economic, ideational, technical, infrastructural, military and fiscal capacities (Nelissen 2002; Cummings and Nørgaard 2004; Savoia and Sen 2012).

In line with this focus on capacity as capabilities and resources, Martin Painter and Jon Pierre have defined policy capacity as "the ability to marshal the necessary resources to make intelligent collective choices about and set strategic directions for the allocation of scare resources to public ends" (Painter and Pierre 2004, p. 2). Painter and Pierre go on to argue that policy capacity is different from administrative capacity or state capacity, where

> Administrative capacity refers to the ability to manage efficiently the human and physical resources required for delivering the outputs of government, while state capacity is a measure of the state's ability to mobilize social and economic support and consent for the achievement of public-regarding goals. (Painter and Pierre 2004, p. 2)

More than simply focusing on human and physical resources or state-society relations, policy capacity in Painter and Pierre's conceptualisation

> draws attention to the structural characteristics and resource stocks of a governing system. The flow of these stocks – that is, the ways in which they are channelled so as to be available when needed – is governed by particular needs and contingencies. They not only have to be created, stored and marshalled, but also put to use. Thus evidence of policy capacity can be gathered both from the analysis of the quality and quantity of institutional resources and from the success of specific outputs and outcomes. (Painter and Pierre 2004, p. 3)

However, Painter and Pierre's definition of policy capacity remains at an overly-broad level of conception. In reality, policymakers and public officers draw on a broad array of skills and resources in their daily work. This includes skills such as accountancy, strategic planning and public relations, among others, as well as resources such as human capital, financial resources, data and knowledge, etc. In other words, there is a need to further breakdown this notion of policy capacity into components that would make sense to the policymaker or public servant on the ground.

A more recent stream of research on policy capacity has sought to understand capacity as the "set of skills and resources—or competences and capabilities—necessary to perform policy functions" (Wu et al. 2015, p. 166). In this body of work, policy capacity is conceptualised in terms of skills and competencies—analytical, operational and political—at the individual, organizational and systemic levels (Wu et al. 2015, 2018). As Wu et al. have further noted, taking this competence-based understanding of policy capacity allows for a broader analysis that covers the entire policy process, rather than a particular policy function or task.

This broad and integrated approach is particularly relevant for the case of Singapore, which has taken on a 'whole-of-government' approach to managing Covid-19. This book therefore draws on this set of research by focusing on analytical, operational and political capacities in Singapore's efforts to manage the Covid-19 pandemic. It also includes a fourth type of capacity, material capacity. This is illustrated in Fig. 2.1.

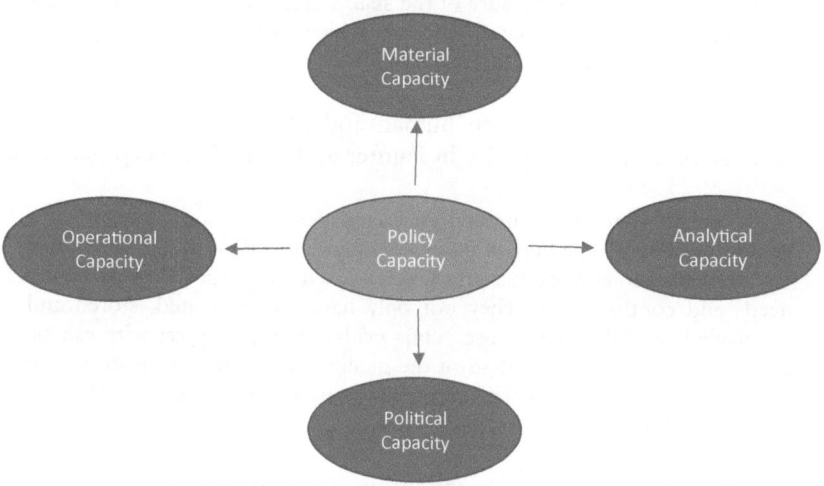

Fig. 2.1   Forms of policy capacity

Material Capacity

The first source of capacity that often comes to mind is material capacity, which has also often been referred to as fiscal capacity by policy analysts and scholars. Material capacity essentially refers to the tangible resources and capabilities that governments can draw upon and apply to a policy problem. There are several types of material capacity that governments typically utilise.

The first of these is financial resources. Also known in economics as 'fiscal space', financial resources allow governments to fund and implement their policy programmes and initiatives. This is particularly important during a crisis, when governments may be required to implement fiscal or monetary stimuli to counteract the economic impacts of a crisis. While a fiscal stimulus would involve drawing upon the government's financial reserves, a monetary stimulus requires the government to mobilise its foreign currency reserves, or at least possess enough of it to keep its financial system liquid.

As I will show in the following chapters, Singapore's response to the SARS and Covid-19 pandemics crises drew heavily from its financial resources. These resources were largely drawn from the government's large current and past reserves and were mostly directed towards supporting the economy through wage subsidies for employers and cash pay-outs for households. Financial resources therefore represent an important set of policy capacities that enable policymakers to implement the policy programmes necessary for crisis management and response.

Aside from financial resources, material capacity also includes other tangible resources such as human capital, technology, urban infrastructure, and the military industrial complex.

In economics, human capital, or labour, is often seen as a critical driver of economic growth (Mincer 1984; Becker et al. 1990; Barro 2001; Barra and Zotti 2017). Labour is a key factor of production in the traditional production function, with land and capital being the other two factors. Aside from driving economic growth, human capital also plays a crucial role in the policy process, with governments relying on public servants as well as other members of society to implement their policies effectively.

As I will show in Chapter 4, Singapore's contact tracing efforts during the Covid-19 pandemic relied heavily on existing public servants as well as personnel from the military and the police force, while volunteers were mobilised to enforce social distancing in its public spaces. In both instances, the availability of an educated and skilled population that could be easily retrained and mobilised for various pandemic response functions contributed to Singapore's Covid-19 response.

Aside from human capital, another form of material capacity is technology. This includes the technological hardware and the broader technology and innovation ecosystem. The importance of technology as a form of material capacity is particularly relevant in 'smart cities' that have sought to develop high-growth technology sectors such as artificial intelligence, big data and the Internet of Things, with such digital technology often also used to enhance policymakers' ability to implement and enforce policies.

In many of these cities, cutting edge digital tools such as artificial intelligence and data analytics have been used to manage Covid-19 infections, particularly through enhancing key policy initiatives such as contact tracing and quarantine surveillance. At the heart of such efforts is a city's technological infrastructure, which can include smart grids, data servers, and a well-developed internet and telecommunications network, among others. The technological firms and public agencies that form a country's technology and innovation ecosystem can also play an important role in developing innovative new solutions for virus testing and patient management

As the experiences of South Korea, Taiwan, Hong Kong and Singapore have shown, cities and countries that possess strong technological infrastructure have proven more capable of managing pandemics such as SARS and Covid-19. Whether it is the application of data analytics and artificial intelligence to contact tracing or the creation of cheaper and faster virus test kits, technological infrastructure and the presence of a technology and innovation cluster are significant sources of material capacity, with technological innovations providing policymakers with possible tools for crisis management.

Indeed, the onset of the Covid-19 had prompted city governments across the world to accelerate their digital transformation efforts through the adoption of smart city technologies (ABI Research 2020). It is also important to note the technology and innovation ecosystem is often driven by public agencies, particularly those from the military.

Defence agencies form an important part of a country's military-industrial complex, which refers to the close network formed by a country's military and the industries that produce military armaments and technology (Wirls 2019). As I will show in Chapter 4, the Singapore

Army, the Defence Science and Technology Agency and government-owned defence technology firm ST Engineering all played crucial roles in supporting the government's Covid-19 response efforts.

Lastly, a country's urban and physical infrastructure can also be seen as a form of material capacity. This is especially the case in city-states such as Hong Kong and Singapore, where limited physical space had led to the conversion of vacant apartment blocks, hotels and convention centres into quarantine facilities for infected persons. Key urban infrastructure such apartment blocks and convention centres are therefore a valuable tangible resource that can be tapped on in the event of a crisis. As I will show in the following chapters, other key urban infrastructure that were mobilised by the Singapore government to deal with Covid-19 also included public transport infrastructure and private-hire vehicles.

Material capacities therefore provide policymakers with an important pool of tangible resources that can be drawn upon, converted and adapted into tools and capacities for dealing with crises. However, material resources alone are not sufficient for effective policymaking and crisis management. As the example of the United States during Covid-19 has shown, even countries with abundant financial resources, urban infrastructure and a large military-industrial complex can struggle with managing a crisis, with American deaths from Covid-19 exceeding 130,000 at time of writing (CNA 2020).

Analytical Capacity

In order to understand why some countries are particularly adept at crisis management, it is necessary to take a step back in the policy process. In other words, there is a need to think about policymaker's abilities to pre-empt and prepare for a crisis before the crisis emerges. This notion of pre-empting, or even predicting, crises is not new. Countries, like business entities, often engage in horizon scanning and risk management activities, in order to predict and prevent potential threats and crises.

Such activities require what is known as analytical capacity. Defined as the knowledge and skills required for effective policy analysis and evaluation, analytical capacity refers to the ability of individuals and organisations to diagnose policy problems and their root causes and evaluate the range of possible policy solutions that can be applied to resolve these policy problems (Wu et al. 2018, p. 6). In traditional public policy theory, analytical capacity is associated with the 'agenda-setting' stage of the policy process, whereby policy problems are first identified and defined.

At this agenda-setting stage, policymakers should theoretically be able to establish clear definitions of policy problems, based on the various channels through which a policy issue could emerge on policymakers' agenda, whether these are in-house researchers, the media or the general public (Kingdon 1984; Baumgartner and Jones 1993; Walgrave et al. 2008). However, the reality is often much more complex. As later chapters will show, policymakers can often be blindsided by policy problems that they are unaware of.

Known as 'black swan' events, such policy problems tend to be highly complex and typically exact a heavy cost on society, even such black swan events do not occur frequently (Ho 2008; Taleb 2010). In light of such black swan events, governments across the world have sought to develop tools that allow them to predict future policy problems and issues, with the aim of establishing the resources and capacities needed for addressing such problems, before they actually occur. These tools include strategic foresight, horizon scanning, risk assessment and scenario planning.

Strategic foresight and scenario planning activities are typically carried out by specialised futures units that are established within the government, with the United Kingdom, Finland, Singapore and the Netherlands seen as leading proponents of government foresight (Varelius et al. 2002; Habegger 2010). Strategic foresight therefore represents an increasingly important form of analytical capacity, with government 'futurists' often trained in a specific set of tools and methodologies that allow them to carry out effective scenario planning and strategic foresight activities (Higgott and Woo 2019).

It is therefore now clear that there are two components of analytical capacity, one that is focused on the present and another that is focused on the future. While futures and foresight units are increasingly useful forms of analytical capacity that can be applied to the identification and definition of future policy problems, it is also important to focus on developing analytical capacity for the present. Such capacities are important for identifying policy problems that emerge in real time, and which may have slipped through the cracks of the futures and foresight analysis.

A growing body of research on 'evidence-based policymaking' has emerged to address this need for real-time policy analysis, with much of this work focused on the use of data and information ('evidence') as inputs into the policy and decision-making process, with the aim of improving the accuracy and efficacy of policy decisions (Sanderson 2002; Head 2008; Howlett 2009; Cartwright and Hardie 2012). However, evidence-based policy can also often result in biased decisions, with the choice of empirical data-sets and experts often a influenced by political variables (Head 2013; Cairney 2016).

Aside from evidence-based policy, policy scholars have also called for a greater role of policy analysts within government (Olejniczak et al. 2018). Employed as civil servants within public agencies, these policy analysts are often tasked with information-related roles such as collecting, interpreting and analysing data, developing policy proposals based on such data, and drafting up policy reports that can be used as a guide for policymaking by senior policymakers and political leaders.

At the organisational level, analytical capacity can be developed by constant training and updating of public servants' ability to identify and define policy problems. In many instances, dedicated schools of public policy or civil service training centres can be useful avenues through which public servants can be trained and re-skilled in the art of problem definition. Many policy schools across the world play this function through their executive education courses, with public servants often incentivised, or even mandated, to attend periodic public policy executive education courses.

Lastly, analytical capacity also includes the technological tools and aids that can be used to rapidly analyse large volumes of data and help policymakers develop a clearer understanding of the problem at hand. Such tools include data analytics, sensors, artificial intelligence, and even social media. These tools allow policymakers to collect large amounts of data—such as demographic data, traffic information, GPS locational data of citizens, and online social sentiments—and incorporate these into their policy formulation and decision-making processes.

As reports by Deloitte have shown, the Singapore government has utilised data analytics to enhance its organisational operations and public service delivery mechanisms across its various ministries and departments (Deloitte 2015, 2020). My discussions in Chapter 4 will also show the key role played by data analytics and GPS locational information in the Singapore government's contact tracing efforts. Analytical capacity therefore represents an important set of resources and competencies for any government, allowing policymakers to make sense of the situation at hand and providing them with the necessary data and information for making more accurate and effective policies.

Operational Capacity

Having collected processed the relevant data and information, the next step of the policy process typically involves translating this data into actionable policies and, ultimately, implementing these policies. Hence aside from analytical capacity, governments also need to build up the operational capacities that are necessary for the day-to-day functioning of government. Operational capacity involves possessing the necessary skills and expertise in various organisational functions, including but not limited to strategic planning, organisational staffing, budgeting, delegation of tasks, directing of policy activities, coordinating across agencies, enforcement of rules and policies, etc. (Wu et al. 2018, pp. 7–8).

In the public policy and public administration literature, it is common to group all these tasks under broader managerial functions, such as leadership, strategic planning and management, public finance, etc. Certainly, much has been said about these various managerial and operational functions. However, it is important to note that our existing understanding of public management and administration remain in a constant state of flux and evolution.

For instance, early understandings of public administration at this operational level tended to draw on the work of Max Weber, who argued that the most efficient bureaucracies tend to be highly hierarchical, with individuals rewarded and promoted on the basis of individual merit (Weber 1919; Evans and Rauch 1999). Known as Weberian bureaucracy, such a hierarchy- and merit-based approach to designing public administration remains relevant, with Singapore often described as a 'neo-Weberian' state due to its hierarchical and highly disciplined civil service (Tan 2008; Quah 2010). However, not all governments subscribe to the Weberian ideal, nor do all public policy scholars endorse this approach.

Beginning the 1990s and spanning through the 2000s, a shift in public administration thinking had placed greater emphasis on the notion of 'governance', which involves states collaborating with non-state actors and organisations in the delivery of public services (Rhodes 1996; Nelissen 2002). This has also sparked off massive governmental privatisation and decentralisation in many developed countries, with policy functions often outsources or contracted out in a movement known as "New Public Management" (NPM) (Hood 1991, 1995; Osborne and Gaebler 1993).

At the heart of these shifts and movements in public administration is the question: how should governments be run? Whether in a hierarchical Weberian bureaucracy or a nimbler NPM-styled administration, the focus has always been on ensuring that the government delivers its public services effectively and efficiently. Taking an operational capacity approach therefore cuts across all these different theoretical approaches by focusing on the specific skills and resources that public agencies and administrators can draw on to carry out their duties.

As was the case with analytical capacity, training and education plays an important role in ensuring that public servants possess the skills and competencies necessary for carrying out their roles. This requires constant training and re-training of public servants, especially with regards to functional skillsets such as financial management, strategic planning and logistics, among others.

Aside from individual skills and expertise, operational capacity also involves organisational structures and institutional forms. These include clarity of organisational mission and individual roles, systems of performance measurement, human resource management, inter-agency division of labour, as well as an organisational culture that both emphasizes discipline and cohesiveness. Much has been written about these variables in both the public administration and business management literature, and there is no need to repeat these here, aside from pointing readers towards the relevant literatures that are listed out in the end-notes of this chapter (Wilkinson and Leggett 1985; Lengnick-Hall and Lengnick-Hall 1988; Hood 1991, 1995; Allison 1992; Palmer 1993; Holzer and Yang 2004; Pollitt and Bouckaert 2011).

In short, a government's success in managing crises and achieving its desired policy outcomes hinges very much on the ability of its bureaucracy and public officers to ensure the smooth and efficient delivery of public services on a day-to-day basis. This requires operational capacity, which in turn is derived from the presence of clearly-defined organisational roles and functions, the operational and managerial skills of policymakers and public officers, as well as enabling organisational cultures such as transparency and a low tolerance for corruption.

Political Capacity

The term 'politics' can be traced back to the ancient Greek word 'politeia', which is in turn related to another Greek word, 'polis'. Made fashionable by the works of the Greek philosophers Plato and Aristotle, polis refers to the city or city-state while politeia encompasses the broad range of social, political and legal relationships involved in the governing of a city. Hence despite its modern-day connotations of elections and ideologies, the nature and activity of politics was initially conceived of as a means through which a city could be governed.

In this section, as well as in the rest of this book, I will draw upon this understanding of politics as the art of governing the city, particularly the socio-political and legal relations that underpin such a governance-centric understanding of politics. Seen in this light, political capacity can then be thought of as the governing competencies and resources needed among political leaders, public agencies and policymakers in order that their policies possess the necessary public support and legitimacy for policy success (Woo et al. 2015; Wu et al. 2015).

As was the case with the previous three capacities, political capacity can be broken down into several driving forces and factors. At the heart of political capacity is the level of socio-political trust that political leaders and policymakers are able to build up with their citizens. This trust is typically exercised within the political, economic, social and security spheres, with policymakers and political leaders applying their political competencies and drawing on institutional and ideational resources to foster trust with citizens across these four spheres (Woo et al. 2015). This in turn allows policymakers to enhance the legitimacy of their policies and ensure compliance from the general public.

Policy scholars have found political trust, and the public support that it connotes, to be an essential prerequisite for effective policy implementation (Weatherford 1989; Woo 2015; Wan et al. 2017). Trust is therefore a resource that governments need to build up, in order that their efforts at crisis management and policy implementation receive the necessary public support and compliance. There are several ways to build up political trust. First of all, transparent legal and political processes, such as democratic elections or fair judges, are necessary for assuring citizens of governmental accountability (Grimes 2006; Font and Blanco 2007; Fukuyama 2011; Zhai 2019). Second, government performance has been seen as a possible contributing factor to a government's efforts to build up trust (Weatherford 1987, 1989).

In many East Asian developmental states, economic performance is a key driver of 'performance legitimacy', with governments building up political trust and legitimacy by promising and ensuring continued economic growth for its citizens (Leftwich 1995; Zhu 2011; Chu 2016; Woo 2018). There is therefore a certain extent of circularity in this trust-performance relationship, with trust being a crucial ingredient for enhancing policy performance but citizens at the same time more willing to trust governments that are capable of ensuring policy and economic performance.

In any case, policy performance can be a means through which political trust and capacity can be built up. This means that the other three capacities that were discussed earlier can contribute to political capacity as well, since the presence of those capacities can in themselves contribute to policy success and performance. Another driver of political trust that policy scholars frequently write about is social capital. This was largely popularised by the work of the political scientist Robert Putnam, who observed that socio-political trust tends to be higher in contexts where there are more civic organisations and institutions, such as religious organisations, guilds and associations (Putnam 1993, 2001).

This central importance of community organisations in turn suggests a need for governments to establish the necessary conditions and frameworks within which civil society and grassroots organisations can thrive and flourish, in the process contributing to the social capital of a country (Maloney et al. 2000; Newton 2001; Keele 2007; Soon and Koh 2017). There is therefore sometimes a paradoxical need for the state to cede some governing and discursive space to non-state actors and organisations, in order to enhance its political capacity. This alludes to the more complex nature of political capacity vis-à-vis the other capacities.

It is also important to note that political capacity can exist at the organisational and individual levels. At these micro- and meso-levels, political capacity requires specific skillsets such as political communication and public relations. Defined by leading political communications scholar Pippa Norris as the "interactive process concerning the transmission of information among politicians, the news media, and the public" (Norris 2001), political communications is a two-way process that includes the 'downward' transmission of key political and policy information from governments to citizens as well as an 'upward' movement of public opinion and ground-level information from citizens to policymakers.

As scholars of political communications have long pointed out, the rapid expansion of new media platforms such as online forums and social media has radically changed the political communications practice and landscape (Norris and Norris 2000; Soon and Kluver 2007; Gurevitch et al. 2009; Soon and Cho 2011; Norris and Reddick 2013). Nonetheless, political communication remains essential for ensuring the efficient and effective transmission of accurate policy information in real-time. This is particularly crucial in times of crisis, where insufficient or ineffective policy communications can give rise to mass panic and irrational behaviour among the public.

This was evident in the mass buying and hoarding of medical equipment and grocery items that occurred in many countries across the world during the Covid-19 pandemic. Policymakers have long recognised this importance of political communications in ensuring public compliance with policies and maintaining social stability during crises, with governments across the world hiring public communications and public relations experts in the civil service, whether as press secretaries to ministers or to staff public relations and communications departments within public agencies. While once exclusive to the private sector, the public relations function is becoming increasingly relevant to the public sector as well.

In sum, the political capacity of a government depends on, at the systemic level, its ability to maintain and sustain socio-political trust with its citizens and at the organisational and individual level, strong political communications and public relations skills among political leaders and policymakers.

CONCLUSION

In this chapter, I have sought to provide a broad and comprehensive understanding of policy capacity. While political scientists and policy scholars have long tried to understand the nature and basis of state strength and capacity, it is the more recent body of work on policy capacity that I have chosen to draw on for my analyses in the following chapters. While I will discuss policy capacity in Singapore's policy response to the Covid-19 pandemic, it is important to also note that there is a growing body of work on how governments across the world have mobilised their policy capacities, or been hampered by the lack thereof, in their Covid-19 responses (Capano et al. 2020).

For instance, a lack of experience with past pandemics had resulted in insufficient capacity in Italy (Capano 2020) while conversely, Singapore's experience with the 2003 SARS crisis had allowed it to build up the policy capacities necessary for handling the Covid-19 pandemic (Woo 2020). Paradoxically, the Hong Kong government's lack of policy and legitimation capacities were offset by the territory's high level of societal capacity, with the latter contributing to Hong Kong's hitherto success in managing its infection levels (Hartley and Jarvis 2020). Jon Pierre has attributed Sweden's high Covid-19-related fatalities to operational capacity deficiencies, specifically the lack of training and equipment among the public officers who are tasked with managing the impacts of the pandemic (Pierre 2020). In larger countries, considerations of policy capacity can be complicated by the presence of multiple levels government, with the case of the United States showing how fiscal capacity, though in abundance at the federal level, can be misapplied or underutilised at the state level (Rocco et al. 2020).

As this emerging body of work shows, there is much interest in how the presence or lack of policy capacity can impact a government's ability to manage the impacts of the Covid-19 pandemic. Such insights can also help governments understand the forms of capacities that will need to be built up in anticipation of future pandemics and policy crises. In the rest of this book, I will discuss the policy capacities that have contributed to Singapore's success efforts to contain the SARS and Covid-19 pandemics.

REFERENCES

ABI Research. (2020). *COVID-19 to Accelerate Adoption of Technology-Enabled Smart Cities Resilience Approaches: Robotics, Digital Twins, and Autonomous Freight* [online]. Available from: https://www.abiresearch.com/press/covid-19-accelerate-adoption-technology-enabled-smart-cities-resilience-approaches-robotics-digital-twins-and-autonomous-freight/. Accessed 14 July 2020.

Allison, G. T. (1992). Public and Private Management: Are They Fundamentally Alike in All Unimportant Respects? In G. M. Shafritz & A. C. Hyde (Eds.), *Classics of Public Administration* (pp. 457–474). Belmont, CA: Wordsworth.

Bakvis, H. (2000). Rebuilding Policy Capacity in the Era of the Fiscal Dividend: A Report from Canada. *Governance, 13*(1), 71–103.

Barra, C., & Zotti, R. (2017). Investigating the Human Capital Development–Growth Nexus, Investigating the Human Capital Development–growth Nexus: Does the Efficiency of Universities Matter?, Does the Efficiency of Universities Matter? *International Regional Science Review, 40*(6), 638–678.

Barro, R. J. (2001). Human Capital and Growth. *American Economic Review, 91*(2), 12–17.

Baumgartner, F. R., & Jones, B. D. (1993). *Agendas and Instability in American Politics.* Chicago: University of Chicago Press.

Becker, G. S., Murphy, K. M., & Tamura, R. (1990). Human Capital, Fertility, and Economic Growth. *Journal of Political Economy, 98*(5, Part 2), S12–S37.

Besley, T., & Persson, T. (2008). Wars and State Capacity. *Journal of the European Economic Association, 6*(2–3), 522–530.

Bräutigam, D., & Xiaoyang, T. (2012). Economic Statecraft in China's New Overseas Special Economic Zones: Soft Power, Business or Resource Security? *International Affairs, 88*(4), 799–816.

Cairney, P. (2016). *The Politics of Evidence-Based Policy Making*. London, UK: Palgrave Macmillan.

Capano, G. (2020). Policy Design and State Capacity in the COVID-19 Emergency in Italy: If You Are Not Prepared for the (Un)Expected, You Can Be Only What You Already Are. *Policy and Society, 39*(3), 326–344.

Capano, G., Howlett, M., Jarvis, D. S. L., Ramesh, M., & Goyal, N. (2020). Mobilizing Policy (In)Capacity to Fight COVID-19: Understanding Variations in State Responses. *Policy and Society, 39*(3), 285–308.

Cartwright, N., & Hardie, J. (2012). *Evidence-Based Policy: A Practical Guide to Doing It Better* (1st ed.). Oxford, U.K.: Oxford University Press.

Chibber, V. (2002). Bureaucratic Rationality and the Developmental State. *American Journal of Sociology, 107*(4), 951–989.

Chong, A. (2010). Small State Soft Power Strategies: Virtual Enlargement in the Cases of the Vatican City State and Singapore. *Cambridge Review of International Affairs, 23*(3), 383–405.

Chu, Y. (2016). The Asian Developmental State: Ideas and Debates. In Y. Chu (Ed.), *The Asian Developmental State* (pp. 1–25). New York: Palgrave Macmillan.

CNA. (2020). *US COVID-19 Outbreak Soon to Be Deadlier Than Any Flu Since 1967* [online]. CNA. Available from: https://www.channelnewsasia.com/news/world/covid-19-coronavirus-outbreak-deadlier-flu-1967-12689872. Accessed 1 May 2020.

Cummings, S. N., & Nørgaard, O. (2004). Conceptualising State Capacity: Comparing Kazakhstan and Kyrgyzstan. *Political Studies, 52*(4), 685–708.

Cutler, A. C. (2003). *Private Power and Global Authority: Transnational Merchant Law in the Global Political Economy*. Cambridge: Cambridge University Press.

Cutler, A. C., Haufler, V., & Porter, T. (1999). *Private Authority and International Affairs*. Albany: State University of New York Press.

Deloitte. (2015). *Smart Governance in a Smart Nation A Singapore Perspective*. Deloitte.

Deloitte. (2020). *Analytics for the Singapore Government* [online]. Deloitte Singapore. Available from: https://www2.deloitte.com/sg/en/pages/public-sector/articles/ps-analytics-singapore.html. Accessed 2 May 2020.

Douglass, M. (1994). The 'Developmental State' and the Newly Industrialised Economies of Asia. *Environment and Planning a, 26*(4), 543–566.

Evans, P., & Rauch, J. E. (1999). Bureaucracy and Growth: A Cross-National Analysis of the Effects of 'Weberian' State Structures on Economic Growth. *American Sociological Review, 64*(5), 748–765.

Evans, P. B. (1989). Predatory, Developmental, and Other Apparatuses: A Comparative Political Economy Perspective on the Third World State. *Sociological Forum, 4*(4), 561–587.

Evans, P. B. (1995). *Embedded Autonomy: States & Industrial Transformation* (1st ed.). Princeton, NJ: Princeton University Press.

Evans, P. B. (2014). The Capability Enhancing Developmental State: Concepts and National Trajectories. In E. M. Kim & P. H. Kim (Eds.), *The South Korean Development Experience* (pp. 83–110). London, UK: Palgrave Macmillan.

Fearon, J., & Laitin, D. (2003). Ethnicity, Insurgency, and Civil War. *American Political Science Review, 97*(1), 75–90.

Font, J., & Blanco, I. (2007). Procedural Legitimacy and Political Trust: The Case of Citizen Juries in Spain. *European Journal of Political Research, 46*(4), 557–589.

Fukuyama, F. (2011). *The Origins of Political Order: From Prehuman Times to the French Revolution*. New York, NY: Farrar, Straus and Giroux.

Ganesan, N. (2005). *Realism and Dependence in Singapore's Foreign Policy*. London: Routledge.

Grimes, M. (2006). Organizing Consent: The Role of Procedural Fairness in Political Trust and Compliance. *European Journal of Political Research, 45*(2), 285–315.

Guo, Y., & Woo, J. J. (2016). *Singapore and Switzerland: Secrets to Small State Success*. Hackensack, NJ: World Scientific Publishing.

Gurevitch, M., Coleman, S., & Blumler, J. G. (2009). Political Communication—Old and New Media Relationships. *The ANNALS of the American Academy of Political and Social Science, 625*(1), 164–181.

Habegger, B. (2010). Strategic Foresight in Public Policy: Reviewing the Experiences of the UK, Singapore, and the Netherlands. *Futures, 42*(1), 49–58.

Hameiri, S. (2007). Failed States or a Failed Paradigm? State Capacity and the Limits of Institutionalism. *Journal of International Relations and Development, 10*(2), 122–149.

Hartley, K., & Jarvis, D. S. L. (2020). Policymaking in a Low-Trust State: Legitimacy, State Capacity, and Responses to COVID-19 in Hong Kong. *Policy and Society, 39*(3), 403–423.

Haufler, V. (2001). *A Public Role for the Private Sector: Industry Self-Regulation in a Global Economy*. Washington: Carnegie Endowment for International Peace.

Head, B. W. (2008). Three Lenses of Evidence-Based Policy. *Australian Journal of Public Administration, 67*(1), 1–11.

Head, B. W. (2013). Evidence-Based Policymaking—Speaking Truth to Power? *Australian Journal of Public Administration, 72*(4), 397–403.

Hellmann, O. (2018). High Capacity, Low Resilience: The 'Developmental' State and Military–Bureaucratic Authoritarianism in South Korea. *International Political Science Review, 39*(1), 67–82.

Higgott, R., & Woo, J. J. (2019). International Political Economy: A Global 'Policy Turn'? In D. Stone & K. Moloney (Eds.), *The Oxford Handbook of Global Policy and Transnational Administration* (pp. 310–327). Oxford, UK: Oxford University Press.

Ho, P. (2008). *Governing at the Leading Edge: Black Swans, Wild Cards, and Wicked Problems*.

Holsti, K. J., & Holsti, K. J. (1996). *The State, War, and the State of War*. Cambridge, UK: Cambridge University Press.

Holt, J., & Manning, N. (2014). *Fukuyama Is Right About Measuring State Quality: Now What?* Governance, Research Note.

Holzer, M., & Yang, K. (2004). Performance Measurement and Improvement: An Assessment of the State of the Art. *International Review of Administrative Sciences, 70*(1), 15–31.

Hood, C. (1991). A Public Management for All Seasons? *Public Administration, 69*(1), 3–19.

Hood, C. (1995). The "New Public Management" in the 1980s: Variations on a Theme. *Accounting, Organizations and Society, 20*(2–3), 93–109.

Howlett, M. (2009). Policy Analytical Capacity and Evidence-Based Policy-Making: Lessons from Canada. *Canadian Public Administration, 52*(2), 153–175.

Howlett, M., & Lejano, R. P. (2013). Tales From the Crypt The Rise and Fall (and Rebirth?) of Policy Design. *Administration & Society, 45*(3), 357–381.

Howlett, M., & Lindquist, E. (2004). Policy Analysis and Governance: Analytical and Policy Styles in Canada. *Journal of Comparative Policy Analysis: Research and Practice, 6*(3), 225–249.

Howlett, M., Mukherjee, I., & Woo, J. J. (2015). From Tools to Toolkits in Policy Design Studies: The New Design Orientation and Policy Formulation Research. *Policy and Politics, 43*(2), 291–311.

Johnson, C. A. (1982). *MITI and the Japanese Miracle: The Growth of Industrial Policy, 1925–1975* (1st ed.). Stanford, CA: Stanford University Press.

Keele, L. (2007). Social Capital and the Dynamics of Trust in Government. *American Journal of Political Science, 51*(2), 241–254.

Kingdon, J. W. (1984). *Agendas, Alternatives, and Public Policies*. Boston: Brown Little.

Krasner, S. D. (1976). State Power and the Structure of International Trade. *World Politics, 28*(03), 317–347.

Lee, G. (2009). A Theory of Soft Power and Korea's Soft Power Strategy. *Korean Journal of Defense Analysis, 21*(2), 205–218.

Leftwich, A. (1995). Bringing Politics Back In: Towards a Model of the Developmental State. *Journal of Development Studies, 31*(3), 400–427.

Leifer, M. (2000). *Singapore's Foreign Policy: Coping with Vulnerability*. London: Routledge.

Lengnick-Hall, C. A., & Lengnick-Hall, M. L. (1988). Strategic Human Resources Management: A Review of the Literature and a Proposed Typology. *The Academy of Management Review, 13*(3), 454–470.

Lim, M. Z. (2020). Wuhan Virus: SAF Working Round the Clock to Ensure 5.2m Masks to Be Given Out Are Packed by Saturday [online]. *The Straits Times*. Available from: https://www.straitstimes.com/singapore/wuhan-virus-saf-working-round-the-clock-to-ensure-52m-masks-to-be-given-out-are-packed-by. Accessed 25 April 2020.

Mahmud, A. H. (2020). *SAF Making Thousands of Calls a Day to Contact Trace, Check Stay-Home Compliance as COVID-19 Fight Hits 'Critical Juncture'* [online]. CNA. Available from: https://www.channelnewsasia.com/news/singapore/saf-contact-trace-stay-home-notice-shn-covid-19-12606752. Accessed 25 April 2020.

Maloney, W., Smith, G., & Stoker, G. (2000). Social Capital and Urban Governance: Adding a More Contextualized 'Top-down' Perspective. *Political Studies, 48*(4), 802–820.

Mincer, J. (1984). Human Capital and Economic Growth. *Economics of Education Review, 3*(3), 195–205.

Mukherjee, I., & Bali, A. S. (2019). Policy Effectiveness and Capacity: Two Sides of the Design Coin. *Policy Design and Practice, 2*(2), 103–114.

Nelissen, N. (2002). The Administrative Capacity of New Types of Governance. *Public Organization Review, 2*(1), 5–22.

Newton, K. (2001). Trust, Social Capital, Civil Society, and Democracy. *International Political Science Review, 22*(2), 201–214.

Norris, D. F., & Reddick, C. G. (2013). Local E-Government in the United States: Transformation or Incremental Change? *Public Administration Review, 73*(1), 165–175.

Norris, P. (2001). Political Communication. In N. J. Smelser & P. B. Baltes (Eds.), *International Encyclopedia of the Social & Behavioral Sciences* (pp. 11631–11640). Oxford: Elsevier.

Norris, P., & Norris, M. L. in C.P.P. (2000). *A Virtuous Circle: Political Communications in Postindustrial Societies*. Cambridge, UK: Cambridge University Press.

Nye, J. S. (2005). *Soft Power: The Means to Success in World Politics* (New ed.). New York: Public Affairs.

Olejniczak, K., Sliwowski, P., & Trzcinski, R. (2018). The Role of Analysts in Public Agencies: Toward an Empirically Grounded Typology. In *Policy Capacity and Governance: Assessing Governmental Competencies and Capacities in Theory and Practice* (pp. 151–178). London: Palgrave Macmillan.

Osborne, D., & Gaebler, T. (1993). *Reinventing Government: How the Entrepreneurial Spirit Is Transforming the Public Sector*. New York, NY: Plume.

Painter, M., & Pierre, J. (2004). *Challenges to State Policy Capacity: Global Trends and Comparative Perspectives*. London: Palgrave Macmillan.

Painter, M., & Pierre, J. (2005). Unpacking Policy Capacity: Issues and Themes. In M. Painter & J. Pierre (Eds.), *Challenges to State Policy Capacity: Global Trends and Comparative Perspectives* (pp. 1–18). Basingstoke: Palgrave Macmillan.

Palmer, A. J. (1993). Performance Measurement in Local Government. *Public Money & Management, 13*(4), 31–36.

Parsons, W. (2004). Not Just Steering but Weaving: Relevant Knowledge and the Craft of Building Policy Capacity and Coherence. *Australian Journal of Public Administration, 63*(1), 43–57.

Perraton, J. (2005). What's Left of 'State Capacity'? The Developmental State After Globalization and the East Asian Crisis. In G. Harrison (Ed.), *Global Encounters: International Political Economy, Development and Globalization* (pp. 95–113). London: Palgrave Macmillan.

Pierre, J. (2020). Nudges Against Pandemics: Sweden's COVID-19 Containment Strategy in Perspective. *Policy and Society, 39*(3), 478–493.

Pollitt, C., & Bouckaert, G. (2011). *Public Management Reform: A Comparative Analysis—New Public Management, Governance, and the Neo-Weberian State* (3rd ed.). Oxford and New York: Oxford University Press.

Putnam, R. D. (1993). *Making Democracy Work: Civic Traditions in Modern Italy*. Princeton, NJ: Princeton University Press.

Putnam, R. D. (2001). *Bowling Alone: The Collapse and Revival of American Community* (1st ed.). New York: Simon & Schuster.

Quah, J. S. T. (2010). *Public Administration Singapore-Style*. Singapore: Emerald Group Publishing.

Ramesh, M. (1995). Economic Globalization and Policy Choices. *Governance: An International Journal of Policy and Administration, 8*(2), 243–260.

Rhodes, R. A. W. (1996). The New Governance: Governing Without Government. *Political Studies, 44*(4), 652–667.

Rocco, P., Béland, D., & Waddan, A. (2020). Stuck in Neutral? Federalism, Policy Instruments, and Counter-Cyclical Responses to COVID-19 in the United States. *Policy and Society, 39*(3), 458–477.

Rotberg, R. I. (2002). Failed States in a World of Terror. *Foreign Affairs, 81,* 127.

Sanderson, I. (2002). Evaluation, Policy Learning and Evidence-Based Policy Making. *Public Administration, 80*(1), 1–22.

Savoia, A., & Sen, K. (2012). *Measurement and Evolution of State Capacity: Exploring a Lesser Known Aspect of Governance* (ESID Working Paper No. 10). Manchester, UK: Effective States and Inclusive Development Research Centre (ESID).

Seabrooke, L. (2002). *Bringing Legitimacy Back Into Neo-Weberian State Theory and International Relations.*

Skocpol, T., & Finegold, K. (1982). State Capacity and Economic Intervention in the Early New Deal. *Political Science Quarterly, 97*(2), 255–278.

Soon, C., & Cho, H. (2011). Flows of Relations and Communication Among Singapore Political Bloggers and Organizations: The Networked Public Sphere Approach. *Journal of Information Technology & Politics, 8*(1), 93–109.

Soon, C., & Kluver, R. (2007). The Internet and Online Political Communities in Singapore. *Asian Journal of Communication, 17*(3), 246–265.

Soon, C., & Koh, G. (Eds.). (2017). *Civil Society and the State in Singapore.* London: World Scientific Europe.

Sørensen, G. (1993). Democracy, Authoritarianism and State Strength. *The European Journal of Development Research, 5*(1), 6–34.

Strange, S. (1996). *The Retreat of the State: The Diffusion of Power in the World Economy.* Cambridge: Cambridge University Press.

Taleb, N. N. (2010). *The Black Swan: Second Edition: The Impact of the Highly Improbable: With a New Section: 'On Robustness and Fragility'* (2nd ed.). New York: Random House Trade Paperbacks.

Tan, K. P. (2008). Meritocracy and Elitism in a Global City: Ideological Shifts in Singapore. *International Political Science Review/Revue internationale de science politique, 29*(1), 7–27.

Taylor, B. D., & Botea, R. (2008). Tilly Tally: War-Making and State-Making in the Contemporary Third World. *International Studies Review, 10*(1), 27–56.

Tee, Z. (2020). Coronavirus: 'Fast' Teams in Place at All 43 Dormitories to Tackle Situation [online]. *The Straits Times.* Available from: https://www.straitstimes.com/singapore/fast-teams-in-place-at-all-43-dormitories-to-tackle-situation. Accessed 25 April 2020.

Varelius, J., Marttinen, J., & Kaivo-oja, J. (2002). Basic Conceptions and Visions of the Regional Foresight System in Finland. *Foresight, 4*(6), 34–45.

Volgy, T. J., & Bailin, A. (2003). *International Politics & State Strength.* London: Lynne Rienner Publishers.

Walgrave, S., Soroka, S., & Nuytemans, M. (2008). The Mass Media's Political Agenda-Setting Power: A Longitudinal Analysis of Media, Parliament, and Government in Belgium (1993 to 2000). *Comparative Political Studies, 41*(6), 814–836.

Waltz, K. N. (1954). *Man, the State, and War: A Theoretical Analysis*. New York, NY: Columbia University Press.

Wan, C., Shen, G. Q., & Choi, S. (2017). A Review on Political Factors Influencing Public Support for Urban Environmental Policy. *Environmental Science & Policy, 75*, 70–80.

Wang, Y. (2008). Public Diplomacy and the Rise of Chinese Soft Power. *The ANNALS of the American Academy of Political and Social Science, 616*(1), 257–273.

Weatherford, M. S. (1987). How Does Government Performance Influence Political Support? *Political Behavior, 9*(1), 5–28.

Weatherford, M. S. (1989). Political Economy and Political Legitimacy: The Link Between Economic Policy and Political Trust. In H. D. Clarke, M. C. Stewart, & G. Zuk (Eds.), *Economic Decline and Political Change: Canada, Great Britain, and the United States* (pp. 225–252). Pittsburgh, PA: University of Pittsburgh Press.

Weber, M. (1919). Politics as a Vocation. In H. H. Gerth & C. W. Wright (Eds.), *From Max Weber: Essays in Sociology* (pp. 77–128). New York, NY: Oxford University Press.

Weiss, L. (1998). *The Myth of the Powerless State*. Ithaca, NY: Cornell University Press.

Weiss, L. (2000). Globalization and State Power. *Development and Society, 29*(1), 1–15.

Weiss, L., & Hobson, J. (1995). *States and Economic Development: A Comparative Historical Analysis*. Cambridge, MA: Polity.

Wilkinson, B., & Leggett, C. (1985). Human and Industrial Relations in Singapore: The Management of Compliance. *Euro-Asia Business Review, 4*, 9–15.

Wirls, D. (2019). Analysis | Eisenhower Called It the 'Military-Industrial Complex.' It's Vastly Bigger Now [online]. *Washington Post*. Available from: https://www.washingtonpost.com/politics/2019/06/26/eisenhower-called-it-military-industrial-complex-its-vastly-bigger-now/. Accessed 1 May 2020.

Woo, J. J. (2015). Policy Relations and Policy Subsystems: Financial Policy in Hong Kong and Singapore. *International Journal of Public Administration, 38*(8), 553–561.

Woo, J. J. (2018). *The Evolution of the Asian Developmental State: Hong Kong and Singapore*. London: Routledge.

Woo, J. J. (2020). Policy Capacity and Singapore's Response to the COVID-19 Pandemic. *Policy and Society, 39*(3) : 345–362.

Woo, J. J., Ramesh, M., & Howlett, M. (2015). Legitimation Capacity: System-Level Resources and Political Skills in Public Policy. *Policy & Society, 34*(3–4), 271–283.

Woo-Cumings, M. (1999). *The Developmental State.* Ithaca, NY: Cornell University Press.

World Bank. (1997). *The State in a Changing World.* New York, NY: World Bank, World Development Report.

World Bank. (2012). *Collaborating to Improve the Measurement of Results from Support for Governance and Public Sector Management Reforms* (Discussion Note). Washington, DC: World Bank.

World Bank. (2014). *AGI Data Portal* [online]. Available from: https://www. agidata.org/site/#.

Wu, X., Howlett, M., & Ramesh, M. (Eds.). (2018). *Policy Capacity and Governance: Assessing Governmental Competences and Capabilities in Theory and Practice.* London: Palgrave Macmillan.

Wu, X., Ramesh, M., & Howlett, M. (2015). Blending Skill and Resources Across Multiple Levels of Activity: Competences, Capabilities and the Policy Capacities of Government. *Policy & Society, 34*(3–4), 165–171.

Zhai, Y. (2019). Popular Democratic Perception Matters for Political Trust in Authoritarian Regimes. *Politics, 39*(4), 411–429.

Zhu, Y. (2011). "Performance Legitimacy" and China's Political Adaptation Strategy. *Journal of Chinese Political Science, 16*(2), 123–140.

CHAPTER 3

Capacity-Building in a Post-SARS World

Abstract In this chapter, I will discuss capacity-building efforts within the realm of Singapore's healthcare sector. I will focus specifically on the institutional and policy capacities that were established after the 2003 SARS crisis. By delineating and categorising these capacities, this chapter provides a broad overview of Singapore's pandemic response processes and procedures, much of which were established in response to the SARS crisis. This will form an important backdrop for Chapter Four's discussions on Singapore's response to the Covid-19 pandemic.

Keywords SARS · Singapore · Pandemic response · Covid-19

It all began with a chance encounter in a lift lobby. It was late February 2003, and the location was the Hotel Metropole in Mongkok, Hong Kong. It was on the 9th floor of that hotel that a doctor from Guangzhou had a chance encounter with 7 other people, three Singaporean women who were on holiday in Hong Kong, a Hong Kong resident who had gone to visit a friend at the hotel, a 48-year-old American businessman, a 55-year-old man from Vancouver and a 78-year-old woman from Toronto (Goh 2003).

Unbeknownst to the rest, the doctor was already infected with the Severe Acute Respiratory Syndrome (SARS) virus. Nobody will know

49
J. J. Woo, *Capacity-building and Pandemics*,
https://doi.org/10.1007/978-981-15-9453-3_3

for sure how the virus was spread. It could have entered the respiratory airways of the 7 individuals when the doctor sneezed. Perhaps he pressed a lift button after having touched his eyes, nose or mouth, with the other individuals pressing the same lift button and unknowingly introducing the virus into their bodies when they touched their faces after that.

This was how the SARS virus entered Singapore, through the 3 women who had that chance encounter with the doctor from Guangzhou. Like the Covid-19 coronavirus, the SARS virus can spread very rapidly, whether through the air droplets that are expelled when an infected individual sneezes or when someone picks up the virus from a surface that an infected individual had previously touched.

Upon their return, the 3 women were hospitalised for atypical pneumonia between 1 and 3 March. However, one of the women—the youngest of the three—inadvertently sparked off a chain of transmission, with the virus spreading to 22 of her contacts (Chew 2020). An air stewardess named Esther Mok, the patient had received visitors while she was in hospital; her doctors were not yet aware of the exact nature of her illness or its mode of transmission (Lawrence 2003). Among these visitors were Mok's father, mother and pastor, all of whom would subsequently pass away from SARS (Yeoh 2003).

The transmission of the SARS virus from Ms Mok to other individuals was further exacerbated by the fact that she, along with the other two women, was initially warded in a 6-bed open ward, with no barrier infection control (Koay 2020). It was only on 12 March 2003 that the WHO issued a global alert on the outbreak of atypical pneumonia, and the virus officially named SARS on 15 March 2020. By 22 March 2003, Singapore had already reported 44 cases of SARS infections, all of whom were either close contacts of the 3 women or hospital staff who had come into contact with them (Ministry of Health 2003a).

A further 14 cases of infection reported on 24 March 2003 would result in the enactment of the Infectious Diseases Act, which required all contacts of infected SARS patients to be quarantined and isolated at home for a period of 10 days (Ministry of Health 2003b). The Act would subsequently be amended on 24 April to introduce stronger penalties for violators. By the time the virus had died down and Singapore was removed from the WHO's SARS watch list on 30 May 2003, 238 people had been infected with SARS while 33 patients had lost their lives to it.

Of the 238 infections, 5 were identified as 'super spreaders' who had infected the vast majority of the other SARS patients (Centre for Infectious Disease Research and Policy 2003). A 'super spreader' is a term that is commonly used in the study of infectious dieases such as Ebola, rubella and laryngeal tuberculosis to describe individuals who are more likely than other typical infected individuals to infect others (Centre for Infectious Disease Research and Policy 2003). Unlike the Covid-19 pandemic, the SARS crisis can be neatly traced back to these 5 super spreaders.

As I will discuss in the rest of this chapter and the next, Singapore's experience with these SARS super spreaders would come to inform its pandemic response efforts, with contact tracing and patient quarantine playing a central role in its efforts to break the transmission chain of both viruses. Border control measures also played an important role in the two pandemics, since both viruses had initially entered Singapore through 'imported cases' who had entered Singapore through its airport.

I will now discuss the policy initiatives and responses that were implemented to manage and contain the SARS crisis, leaving my discussion of Singapore's Covid-19 response to the next chapter.

Singapore's Response

The SARS prevention and control measures that were implemented in Singapore can be broadly grouped under three categories (James et al. 2006):

1. Community Measures
2. Healthcare System Measures
3. International Measures

While community measures were aimed at minimising the spread and transmission of the SARS virus across the broader community, healthcare system measures were implemented to protect healthcare workers from infection. These healthcare system measures would come to be particularly important since most of the SARS infections occurred within healthcare facilities. Aside from such efforts to curb the transmission of the SARS virus within Singapore's local community, international measures were also implemented to reduce the risk of imported cases who may enter Singapore from abroad.

Driving these three groups of measures is the Ministry of Health's SARS Task Force, which was formed on 15 March 2003 and led by the Ministry's Director of Medical Services, Dr Tan Chorh-Chuan. These measures have been largely successful, with the WHO's Executive Director for Communicable Diseases Dr David Heymann stating that "Singapore's handling of its SARS outbreak has been exemplary"(WHO 2003). I will now discuss each group of measures separately.

Community Measures

The prevention and control measures that were implemented within the community were broadly focused on detecting and isolating possible SARS cases, with the ultimate aim of minimising community transmission of the virus within the general population. These measures were very much made possible the Infectious Diseases Act, which was invoked by the Ministry of Health on 24 March 2003. By making non-compliance with quarantine orders a legal offence, the Infectious Diseases Act provided the necessary legal provisions for the authorities to enforce quarantine orders more effectively.

Home quarantine orders were issued to both recovering SARS patients and their close contacts. For SARS patients, a mandatory 10-day home quarantine was imposed upon their discharge from the hospital. Close contacts of confirmed SARS cases were typically identified through contact tracing, an investigative process that involves contact tracing teams who seek to identify all persons who could have come into close contact with an infected person. Once identified, the close contact would then be quarantined at home for 10 days.

In some instances, SARs cases and their contacts were issued quarantine orders that had to be served out in TTSH. These were typically either suspected SARS cases who had already been admitted into TTSH or close contacts of SARS patients who were hospital patients and staff. Given this importance of quarantine orders in breaking the chain of transmission, contact tracing was therefore an important component of Singapore's SARS community measures that allowed for the quick identification of potential SARS cases.

A contact tracing centre was established within the Ministry of Health that allowed up to 200 officers to identify the close contacts of SARS cases observe potential SARS cases. The components of contact tracing included obtaining all patient movement data during his/her symptomatic phase, identifying all persons who had come into contact with the patient during these movements, and instituting follow-up action on these contacts for a 10-day period (Ooi et al. 2005).

Compliance with home quarantine orders was ensured through various channels. First, public officers from the MOH and National Environment Agency (NEA) would check on quarantined individuals on a daily basis. Second, an electronic picture (ePIC) camera was installed at the home of each contact; individuals would have to appear in front of the ePIC camera each time they were called on the telephone by an officer from the NEA or any other enforcement agency (James et al. 2006, p. 24).

Given the large number of home quarantine orders that were issued, officers from the security agency CISCO were subsequently engaged on 10 April 2003 to assist in the issuing and enforcement of home quarantine orders, freeing up health and environmental agency officers to engage in other SARS-management activities (Ooi et al. 2005). Contact tracing therefore allowed for the rapid identification of the people who may have come into contact with SARS cases, preventing further spread of the virus through these potential secondary cases.

Aside from contact tracing, much effort was also placed on identifying potential SARS cases in the broader community. A very broad definition for suspicious cases was used for the identification of potential SARS cases, including individuals with fever and/or respiratory symptoms, patients with atypical pneumonia with no known cause, or clusters of patients and healthcare workers who were assessed to have been exposed to potential SARS cases (Tan 2003, p. 346).

A community measure that was used to identify potential SARS cases in the community therefore involved screening and monitoring body temperature. Daily temperature-taking was instituted across schools and public institutions, with thermometers issued to households and individuals across Singapore. Students and public officers, including military personnel, were therefore required to take their temperature every day, often several times throughout the day.

Aside from public institutions, organisers of mass public events were also encouraged to screen their attendees for fever prior to entry. This extensive temperature-taking regime in public spaces was greatly facilitated by the development and production of the infrared fever screening system by the government's Defence Science and Technology Agency (DSTA) (Tan et al. 2004). Based on existing military thermal imaging technologies, the Infrared Fever Screening System scans the infrared energy that is emitted by individuals through its cameras and produces a coloured thermograph that shows whether an individual is having a fever or not.

The Infrared Fever Screening System has since been named by Time as one of the best inventions of 2003 (*Time* 2003). More importantly, the Infrared Fever Screening System can be used to screen large numbers of people without having to make direct physical contact with any of them. Not only does this enhance the efficiency of fever screening, but it also serves to protect enforcement officers from infection. Such infrared fever screening systems have since been used extensively in airports, schools, public venues and even workplaces across the world, not only during pandemics but in normal times as well.

As I will show in the next chapter, infrared fever screening systems were also rapidly deployed across hospitals, universities, schools and malls upon the onset of the Covid-19 pandemic. The infrared fever screening systems that were invented and produced by DSTA therefore played a critical role in monitoring and controlling community infection during both the SARS and Covid-19 crises. As I will discuss later in this chapter and in the next, technology serves as a key enabler of effective contact tracing and patient monitoring.

As the SARS crisis worsened, primary and secondary schools, junior colleges and centralised tertiary institutes, as well as after-school enrichment centres were closed from 27 March 2003 to 6 April 2003. The decision to close these educational institutes was aimed at preventing or reducing the spread of SARS among students, many of whom typically interact with each other at close proximity in the classroom and during after-school co-curriculum activities such as sports and music interest groups.

Last and by no means least, the government embarked on an extensive public education campaign by disseminating SARS-related information and health advisories on both traditional mass media and online media. A very tangible example of this were the many posters that were placed in public washrooms, detailing the various steps that should be taken when washing one's hands with soap. While not as intrusive as the other measures, these provided the public with the information and guidance necessary for protecting themselves from possible infections.

While these community measures served to prevent widespread community transmission of the SARS virus, it was also critical that the virus did not enter the community via the healthcare institutions that were at the forefront of the fight against SARS. A set of control and prevention measures were therefore established across Singapore's healthcare institutions, particularly those that were directly involved in identifying and treating SARS patients.

Healthcare System Measures

Given the high numbers of healthcare workers who had become infected, SARS was known as a 'nosocomial' infection. In the medical field, nosocomial refers to an infection that either originated from, or predominantly took place in, a hospital. Of the total probable SARS cases that were detected throughout the outbreak, 78% were acquired in a hospital setting (Tan 2003). This high risk of infection among healthcare workers, hospital patients and visitors prompted the government to place a strong focus on controlling and preventing the spread of the virus within the healthcare system.

Among the healthcare system measures that were implemented, none were more important than the decision on 22 March 2003 to designate Tan Tock Seng Hospital (TTSH) as the central 'SARS hospital'. All patients that were found by primary health clinics and emergency departments to be exhibiting SARS-like symptoms were immediately referred and sent to TTSH. Patients who had already been warded in another hospital but who were subsequently found to be infected with SARS were also transferred to TTSH. While the Communicable Disease Centre (CDC) was also involved in treating SARS patients, its limited size meant that the bulk of SARS cases were handled by TTSH.

This centralisation of SARS cases at TTSH served to limit the spread of the virus across Singapore's healthcare system by reducing the infection risks of healthcare workers in other hospitals and healthcare institutions. As I will show in the next chapter, such efforts to centralise the treatment of infected patients during a pandemic would prompt the government to establish a purpose-built hospital for treating infectious diseases. In any case, the move to make TTSH the 'SARS hospital' would prove prescient. Even with the isolation of SARS cases at TTSH, 40% of Singapore's SARS infections were from healthcare workers (Chew 2020).

Within TTSH and across other hospitals in Singapore, strict infection controls were implemented. These included the mandatory use of personal protective equipment (PPE) such as N95 masks, gloves, gowns and goggles or visors. Hospitals also instituted strict control measures such as limiting visitors, screening all incoming patients for SARS symptoms, monitoring healthcare workers for SARS symptoms, and establishing a 24-hour dedicated private ambulance service to transport all possible SARS cases to TTSH (James et al. 2006, p. 23).

Through its community and healthcare system measures, Singapore was able to minimise the spread of the SARS virus, both within the healthcare system and across broader society. However, these measures were only focused on managing the potential spread of SARS within the domestic population. Given Singapore's position as a global city and major tourist hub, it was also necessary to prevent and limit the spread of the virus from international sources. The third set of control and prevention measures that were implemented therefore focused on this international aspect of SARS.

International Measures

Given that Singapore's first case of SARS had entered the city-state through air travel, much attention was placed on screening for SARS cases at Singapore's border checkpoints. Infrared fever screening systems were therefore installed at Singapore's air, sea and land checkpoints to detect any incoming visitors who were having a fever. Visitors were also required to complete a Health Declaration Card that requires them to report any possible SARS-like symptoms. Individuals who were found to be having SARS-like symptoms were then referred to on-site medical staff for further examination, with suspected SARS cases sent to TTSH for further assessment and treatment (James et al. 2006, p. 24).

All airlines that were operating flights to Singapore were also required to conduct passenger screening at their check-in counters in the departing location (Chew 2020). Fever screening was also carried out in the same way for travellers who were leaving Singapore, with any suspected SARS that were picked up also sent to TTSH for isolation and treatment. Lastly, information exchange and sharing were facilitated with the WHO, through special bilateral agreements with Malaysia and Indonesia, as well as through a multilateral agreement with the ASEAN Plus Three community (comprising the 10 ASEAN countries along with Korean, Japan and China).

These aimed to enhance cross-border contact tracing efforts and facilitated broader regional efforts to minimise the transmission of the SARS virus. As the Covid-19 case will also show, such efforts to manage the cross-border spread of an infectious disease is crucial for bringing infections within the domestic population down, by reducing the risk of 'imported cases' that may enter Singapore through its air, sea and land borders.

As the discussions have thus far shown, Singapore had taken a three-pronged approach to managing the SARS crisis that involved community, healthcare system and international measures. However, it is important to note that these responses were not one-off policy initiatives. Rather, many of these initiatives and measures have become internalised as standard operating procedures (SOPs), especially in the event of a future pandemic, or institutional processes that have been documented and passed down from one generation of healthcare policymakers and workers to the next.

These SOPs and institutional procedures, among other factors, can be thought of as policy capacities that were established in the aftermath of the SARS crisis. I will now proceed to discuss the policy capacities that were established by the Singapore government in the aftermath of the SARS crisis.

Post-SARS Policy Capacities

As the discussion thus far has shown, the SARS crisis had prompted the Singapore government to formulate and implement a broad range of policy initiatives aimed at minimising the transmission and impacts of the virus. These included the establishment of taskforces and committees, development and adaptation of technological tools, and the wide-scale deployment of governmental resources, particularly in the form of manpower and financial resources, among others.

In the rest of this chapter, I will frame these initiatives as policy capacities that were developed in response to the SARS crisis and which, as I will discuss in the next chapter, have also been mobilised and deployed to address the Covid-19 pandemic.

Analytical Capacities

Perhaps the most important set of capacities that were built from Singapore's experience with SARS is analytical capacity. Given the extensive collection and analysis of information that is involved, the establishment of contact tracing processes and procedures (especially those that can quickly be replicated in future crises and pandemics) represents a clear instance of analytical capacity-building. As I had discussed in Chapter 2, analytical capacity fundamentally involves the collection and interpretation of policy-relevant data, with the goal of informing and supporting other policy processes such as policy formulation and decision-making.

At the heart of the analytical capacities that were developed post-SARS is the contact tracing centre that was established in the Ministry of Health and which worked closely with a full-time team at TTSH to collect and analyse the contact data of SARS patients as well as interview suspected SARS cases. The expertise and skills of the contact tracers who formed the contact tracing centre, alongside those who were operating from TTSH, are therefore an important source of analytical capacity for Singapore's pandemic response mechanisms.

Aside from contact tracers, enforcement officers who monitored individuals under quarantine through telephone surveillance and physical visits also represent another source of analytical capacity, since these officers were involved in monitoring and collecting information about potential SARS cases. Singapore's experience and success with contact tracing and monitoring during the SARS crisis therefore allowed it to establish the expertise and procedures necessary for rapid scanning and identification of potential infections during a pandemic.

This ability to collect and analyst vast amounts of contact information, as well as conduct 24-hour monitoring of suspected cases represents a significant set of analytical capacities that requires investigative skills and information processing capabilities. Furthermore, Singapore's experience with SARS also revealed a further need to develop other analytical capacities that, while not required during the SARS crisis, may prove crucial for managing future epidemics and pandemics.

As then-Director of Medical Services and current Chief Health Science Officer Tan Chorh Chuan had noted in the aftermath of the SARS crisis, there was a still need to develop rapid and highly sensitive tests for SARS infections in order to enhance Singapore's ability to detect SARS cases as well as minimise the need for quarantine measures, while the lack of asymptomatic SARS infection and transmission also meant that Singapore may not have been sufficiently prepared for this possibility(Tan 2003, p. 347).

This last point would prove prescient, with the subsequent Covid-19 pandemic involving a large extent of asymptomatic infection and transmission.

Another set of analytical capacities that were developed during the SARS crisis was the development of information technology (IT) systems for diagnosing and categorising SARS cases. While the collection and analysis of information were done manually in the initial stages of the SARS outbreak, more sophisticated IT systems were brought to bear on these tasks in mid- to late-April 2003, greatly enhancing Singapore's contacting tracing as well as quarantine and isolation efforts (Tan 2003, p. 349).

This new SARS IT infrastructure included an Infectious Disease Alert and Clinical Database System that integrates clinical, laboratory and contact tracing information, a contact tracing or case management system that can consolidate information on SARS cases, contact history and home quarantine statuses as well as automatically generate home quarantine order reports and contact listings for external agencies, and an e-Quarantine Management System for better processing and enforcement of home quarantine orders by enforcement agencies (Goh et al. 2006, p. 310).

Based on an existing casualty management system that was used by the Singapore Armed Forces, the DSTA developed a case management system (CMS) that gathered data from hospitals, the MOH, MOE, general practitioners and traditional Chinese medicine (TCM) practitioners to develop a database of information on suspected and confirmed SARS patients and their contact information, to be shared with the relevant agencies for contact tracing and quarantine monitoring purposes (Pan et al. 2005).

These systems would no doubt have formed the foundation for the development of the more sophisticated IT and data analytical tools that were used during the Covid-19 pandemic for the purposes of contact tracing as well as the surveillance and monitoring of individuals under quarantine or stay home notices. Singapore's experience in managing the SARS crisis, especially with regards to the collection and analysis of case information, has therefore allowed it to build up significant analytical capacities that can be, and have been, carried forward and applied in future pandemics and healthcare crises.

Operational Capacities

Aside from analytical capacity, key operational capacities were also developed during the SARS crisis. These include several operational readiness and laboratory safety measures that were established in the midst of

the SARS crisis and which have since been retained or institutionalised. For instance, the MOH was reorganised with the incorporation
of an Operations Group that is tasked with the operational aspects of
outbreak prevention and control, the command and control of medical
resources during a crisis, as well as the coordination of health services and
operations during ordinary times (Goh et al. 2006, p. 310).

Critical to the Operations Group's work are the command, control and
coordination systems that allow for such coordination of medical service
delivery, both during a crisis and in ordinary times. As noted by then-
Director of Medical Services Tan Chorh Chuan, Singapore's success in
containing the SARS epidemic depended on "effective command, control
and coordination systems that ensured that strategies and decisions were
properly implemented" (Tan 2003, p. 347).

This included the Ministerial Committee on SARS that allowed for
cross-Ministry policy coordination as well as an Executive Group that
comprised the Permanent Secretaries of key Ministries and which was
focused on the implementation of control and prevention measures. A
SARS taskforce was also set up on 15 March. Comprising hospital leaders,
infectious disease specialists and other experts, the Taskforce provided the
government with advice on public health measures. These committees and
procedures have since been codified in the MOH's Pandemic Readiness
and Response Plan for Influenza and other Acute Respiratory Diseases
(Ministry of Health 2014).

Taken together, these committees and taskforces allowed for closer
coordination of policy formulation, implementation and enforcement.
As I will discussion in the next Chapter, similar committees and taskforces were established during the Covid-19 pandemic. This means
that the frameworks and institutions that were developed to facilitate
policy implementation during SARS were carried forward to Covid-19,
with the institutionalised inter-agency coordination that these connote
representing a key set of operating capacities.

Aside from these high-level committees, operational capacities were
also built up at the institutional and organisational level. As a study that
was published in the Journal of Hospital Medicine has shown, the "testing
and viral spread control challenges during SARS spawned hospital-system
epidemiology capacity building" (Vidyarthi et al. 2020). These included
developing contingency plans for all healthcare institutions and agencies, regular preparedness exercises and audits, building up a stockpile of
critical medical supplies such as PPE that can last for up to 6 months,

establishing more isolation facilities in all hospitals, and creating new biosafety standards at both the organisational and national levels (Goh et al. 2006, p. 310).

Perhaps most crucial of these moves was the decision to commission a 330-bed National Centre for Infectious Diseases (NCID), which was completed in 2019. The NCID, along with other hospitals' expanded isolation units, would come to play a crucial role in Singapore's efforts to contain the Covid-19 pandemic in 2020. However, in the absence of an infectious disease outbreak, these facilities were typically existed as 'excess capacity' which would only be fully utilised during an outbreak. For instance, the NCID was largely used for research activities, while its laboratories handled the testing needs of food poisoning cases.

As I will discuss in Chapter 5, the availability of isolation facilities in the NCID and other hospitals in Singapore, all of which were rapidly mobilised during the Covid-19 pandemic, suggests a need to build up and set aside excess capacity. While governments across the world had throughout the 1990s and 2000s been focusing on resource optimisation and efficiency, there may be a need for more 'slack' in government capacities and resources, with excess capacities and resources kept read on hand, but not necessarily fully utilised or optimised in ordinary times.

Aside from hospital facilities, laboratories also played a crucial role in the rapid testing of SARS and Covid-19 cases, allowing for the testing and identification of infected persons. This ability to conduct high volumes of tests and provide fast test results persons in turn allows the government to quickly identify and isolate infected persons, minimising the risks of transmission from these individuals. Of particular importance to these laboratories are the biosafety standards that were established in the aftermath of the SARS crisis and which contribute to the safety and continuity of laboratory workers.

Lastly, a three colour-coded alert system was also established for assessing the threat level of an epidemic and the extent of its transmission. This would form the basis of the Disease Outbreak Response System Condition (DORSCON) that would play a crucial role in assessing the Covid-19 threat in 2020. The DORSCON system assesses the current situation of an infectious disease, its level and mode of transmission, its likelihood of arriving in Singapore and its potential impacts on the local community, with the four colour codes—green, yellow, orange and red—signalling the varying severity and level of transmission of an infectious disease (Ministry of Health 2020). Each colour code also provides guidance to the public on potential disruptions to daily life and the steps that should be taken to minimise risks of infection.

At the community level, the extensive temperature monitoring regime that was established across public institutions and public spaces, whether through the use of personal thermometers or infrared fever screening systems, led to the development of the necessary resources, hardware and expertise that can be quickly mobilised in the event of another epidemic.

In short, the procedures and standards that were established during SARS to provide pandemic standard operating procedures (SOPs) and guidance for the healthcare sector as well as the general public constitute an important set of operational capacities that were established in the aftermath of the SARS crisis and which have contributed immensely to Singapore's efforts to contain the Covid-19 pandemic.

Material Capacities

Driving the various operational and analytical capacities that were discussed above are the financial resources that were mobilised to address the SARS crisis. Much of this was drawn from a SG$ 230 million SARS relief package that was introduced on 17 April 2003 (Ministry of Finance 2003). The package included a range of grants and tax rebates for tourism-related industries and the transport sector. While the economic impacts of SARS are much lower than that of Covid-19, the introduction of this SARS relief package reflected the government's recognition of the need for fiscal support during a pandemic.

Also, and unlike the Covid-19 pandemic, the impacts of the SARS crisis on Singapore's healthcare system, particularly its healthcare capacity, were not as intense. This means that the TTSH and CDC possessed sufficient capacity to house and treat SARS patients, while individuals on quarantine were mostly able to serve out their quarantines at home. As I will discuss in the next chapter, the Covid-19 crisis had required Singapore to mobilise a broader range of material capacities, including urban spaces and facilities.

Political Capacities

With regards to political capacity, Singapore's success in managing the SARS crisis has certainly built up a significant amount of political trust between the government and its citizens, especially as it pertains to managing and containing infectious diseases. Indeed, scholars have shown that the successful implementation of control and prevention measures during the SARS crisis was predicated upon high levels of compliance with and support for these measures, even if they involved significant intrusions into the personal privacy and social lives of citizens (Teo et al. 2005).

Central to such high levels of societal compliance is a proactive role of is citizens, whether in terms of exercising social responsibility and complying with prevention measures or fostering ground-up initiatives by civil society. It has been noted that Singapore's success in managing SARS was partly driven by a deep mobilisation of society, with citizens and civil society groups driven by both self-interest and voluntarism (Huat 2006).

The government's successful efforts to contain SARS has also contributed immensely to its political capacity. First, it has managed to further strengthen socio-political trust with citizens. This can be attributed to the efficiency and transparency with which the government had addressed the SARS crisis, especially in terms of information sharing and disclosure by the various taskforces and committees that I had discussed earlier (Case 2004).

These efforts also reflect the government's strengths in public communication, which is in itself a crucial component of political capacity. As I had discussed in Chapter 2, effective political and public communications represent an important source of organisational and institutional political capacity. In the case of SARS, the MOH and the SARS Taskforce, through its frequent press releases, have established clear channels for effective communications on the SARS outbreak and the government's intended responses.

This heightened level of socio-political trust and the government's ability to effectively communicate its policy initiatives and position have in turn driven political capacity in Singapore's efforts to manage subsequent healthcare crises, such as the H1N1 pandemic in 2009, Zika outbreak in 2016 and the Covid-19 pandemic in 2020. In all these crises, strong public cooperation and compliance with the government's prevention and control measures allowed Singapore to respond swiftly to outbreaks of infectious diseases.

The socio-political trust that was build up during the SARS crisis as well as the public communications channels that were established should therefore be seen as important forms of political capacity that have been drawn upon for the effective management of future crises.

CONCLUSION

Having discussed the various policy capacities that were established during the SARS crisis, I will now provide a broad overview of the Covid-19 pandemic in the next chapter. Given the ongoing and rapidly-evolving nature of the Covid-19 crisis, there may well be significant developments that occur after this book has gone to print. Should this be the case, I seek the reader's understanding and certainly hope that the reader can plug these possible gaps in the description in the process of reading this book.

REFERENCES

Case, W. (2004). Singapore In 2003: Another Tough Year. *Asian Survey, 44*(1), 115–120.

Centre for Infectious Disease Research and Policy. (2003). *Most SARS Cases in Singapore Traced to Five 'Super Spreaders'* [online]. CIDRAP, University of Minnesota. Available from: https://www.cidrap.umn.edu/news-perspective/2003/05/most-sars-cases-singapore-traced-five-super-spreaders. Accessed 10 May 2020.

Chew, V. (2020). *Severe Acute Respiratory Syndrome (SARS) Outbreak, 2003 | Infopedia* [online]. Singapore Infopedia. Available from: https://eresources.nlb.gov.sg/infopedia/articles/SIP_1529_2009-06-03.html. Accessed 10 May 2020.

Goh, K., Cutter, J., Heng, B., Ma, S., Koh, B. K. W., Kwok, C., et al. (2006). Epidemiology and Control of SARS in Singapore. *Annals of the Academy of Medicine, Singapore, 35*(5), 301–316.

Goh, L. G. (2003). Reflections on the Singapore SARS Outbreak. *SNA News, 35*(3).

Huat, C. B. (2006). Sars Epidemic and the Disclosure of Singapore Nation. *Cultural Politics, 2*(1), 77–96.

James, L., Shindo, N., Cutter, J., Ma, S., & Chew, S. K. (2006). Public Health Measures Implemented During the SARS Outbreak in Singapore, 2003. *Public Health, 120*(1), 20–26.

Kuay, A. (2020). *What Happened in S'pore During the SARS Outbreak in 2003 & How We Dealt with It, Explained* [online]. Mothership.sg. Available from: https://mothership.sg/2020/02/sars-wuhan-outbreak-explained/. Accessed 10 May 2020.

Lawrence, J. (2003). Sars Victim Who Infected 133 Will Remain in Quarantine [online]. *The Independent*. Available from: http://www.independent.co.uk/

news/science/sars-victim-who-infected-133-will-remain-in-quarantine-114
666.html. Accessed 10 May 2020.
Ministry of Finance. (2003). *Government Unveils $230 Million SARS Relief
Package* [online]. Available from: https://www.mof.gov.sg/newsroom/press-
releases. Accessed 17 July 2020.
Ministry of Health. (2003a). *Enhanced Precautionary Measures to Break SARS
Transmission*. Singapore: Ministry of Health, Press Statement.
Ministry of Health. (2003b). *Update on SARS Cases in Singapore: 24 March
2003*. Singapore: Ministry of Health, Press Release.
Ministry of Health. (2014). *Pandemic Readiness and Response Plan for Influenza
and other Acute Respiratory Diseases*. Singapore: Ministry of Health.
Ministry of Health. (2020). *Being Prepared for a Pandemic* [online]. Avail-
able from: https://www.moh.gov.sg/diseases-updates/being-prepared-for-a-
pandemic. Accessed 13 May 2020.
Ooi, P. L., Lim, S., & Chew, S. K. (2005). Use of Quarantine in the Control of
SARS in Singapore. *American Journal of Infection Control, 33*(5), 252–257.
Pan, S. L., Pan, G., & Devadoss, P. R. (2005). E-Government Capabilities
and Crisis Management: Lessons from Combating SARS in Singapore. *MIS
Quarterly Executive, 4*(4), 385–397.
Tan, C.C. (2003). *National Response to SARS: Singapore*.
Tan, Y. H., Teo, C. W., Ong, E., Tan, B. L., & Soo, M. J. (2004). *Development
and Deployment of Infrared Fever Screening Systems*. Proceedings of SPIE—
The International Society for Optical Engineering.
Teo, P., Yeoh, B. S. A., & Ong, S. N. (2005). SARS in Singapore: Surveillance
Strategies in a Globalising City. *Health Policy, 72*(3), 279–291.
Time. (2003). Best Inventions of 2003—TIME. *Time*.
Vidyarthi, A. R., Bagdasarian, N., Esmaili, A. M., Archuleta, S., Monash, B.,
Sehgal, N. L., et al. (2020). Understanding the Singapore COVID-19 Experi-
ence: Implications for Hospital Medicine. *Journal of Hospital Medicine, 15*(5):
281–283.
WHO. (2003). *Singapore Removed from List of Areas with Local SARS Transmission* [online]. WHO. Available from: https://www.who.int/csr/don/
2003_05_30a/en/. Accessed 12 May 2020.
Yeoh, E.-L. (2003). *Singapore Woman Linked to 100 SARS Cases* [online]. Associated Press. Available from: https://www.ph.ucla.edu/epi/bioter/singapore
womanSARS.html. Accessed 10 May 2020.

CHAPTER 4

Singapore's Response to Covid-19

Abstract This chapter will discuss Singapore's response to the Covid-19 pandemic, focusing in particular on how it has mobilised and adapted its policy capacities to deal with the pandemic. I will also discuss the new capacities that were established this period. In focusing on how policy capacities were drawn upon or created in its Covid-19 response, this chapter will provide readers with an understanding of the various policy capacities that are necessary for responding to pandemics and other healthcare crises, as well as the capacity limitations or deficiencies that may have posed challenges for policymakers.

Keywords Covid-19 · Singapore · Pandemic response · Policy capacity

Like the SARS virus, the Covid-19 coronavirus first entered Singapore through its borders. In this case, it was a 66-year-old Chinese national who had arrived in Singapore from Wuhan on 20 January 2020 and was subsequently tested positive for the virus on 23 January 2020 (Yong 2020a). Singapore would within months experience high rates of infection, with the number of confirmed Covid-19 cases exceeding 55,000 as at time of writing. Such high rates of infection were wholly unexpected, given Singapore's excellent public healthcare system and its reputation as a leading medical hub.

© The Author(s), under exclusive license to Springer Nature
Singapore Pte Ltd. 2021
J. J. Woo, *Capacity-building and Pandemics*,
https://doi.org/10.1007/978-981-15-9453-3_4

These high infection rates therefore raise an important question that will be of interest to policy scholars and practitioners alike: how did such high levels of infection occur in a high capacity country such as Singapore? This question will drive the discussions that form the rest of this chapter. While I will devote much attention to the policy capacities that have underpinned Singapore's successful response to the Covid-19 pandemic, I will also discuss the capacity deficiencies that may have caused such high infection rates.

After the entry of the first Covid-19 case into Singapore, seven more cases of Covid-19 infections would be identified on 28 January, all of whom were Chinese nationals from Hubei. Consequently, travellers with recent travel histories to Hubei were barred from entering Singapore while the government began evacuating Singaporeans from Wuhan on 31 January 2020. As the days went by, more Covid-19 cases were found, although all of them were imported cases, i.e. individuals who had caught the virus elsewhere and brought it with them into Singapore.

It would not be long before community transmission took place, with the first cluster emerging on 4 February 2020 in Yong Thai Hang Medical Hall, a traditional Chinese medicine shop that caters mostly to tourists from China. The cluster had emerged when several employees of the medical hall were infected with the virus after prolonged interactions with a group of travellers from China (Tan et al. 2020). The emergence of more community transmission, particular cases without links to previous cases or travel history to China, would prompt the Singapore government to raise the DORSCON level to orange on 7 February 2020.

As more Covid-19 cases and clusters emerged throughout February, the Singapore government introduced new measures to control the spread of the virus, both domestically and from foreign travellers. I will discuss these at greater length below. The subsequent months would bring forth several grim milestones in the progress of the pandemic in Singapore. On 21 March, Singapore announced its first fatalities from the virus. These were a 75-year-old Singaporean woman and a 64-year-old Indonesian man, both of whom had underlying health conditions and were warded in the intensive care unit (ICU). More fatalities would be announced in the coming months, although Singapore's Covid-19 death rate would remain relatively low, compared to those of other countries.

It was however in early April that a major turning point took place. First, increasing local transmission of the coronavirus prompted the government to announce a 'circuit breaker'. Beginning on 7 April 2020, the circuit breaker imposed an elevated set of safe distancing measures, such as the closure of schools and workplaces, except for essential services and critical economic sector, as well as the limiting of food sales to take-away and delivery (i.e. patrons were no longer allowed to dine in) and retail services to the provision of daily living needs (Ministry of Health 2020a). Initially scheduled to last for a month, the circuit breaker was subsequently extended for another month until 1 June 2020.

A second turning point came with the emergence of Covid-19 clusters across several migrant worker dormitories. Infection levels at these dormitories initially numbered in the hundreds daily but subsequently exceeded 1000 cases a day. Many of the workers living in these dormitories were from the construction industry or were involved in essential services sectors such as cleaning services, food and beverage (F&B), healthcare, and public transport, among others. The main cause of these infection clusters are the cramped and unsanitary conditions of the dormitories, much of it arising from poor management by dormitory operators.

Interviews with residents of these dormitories by researchers and VWOs revealed that many dormitories housed 12–20 men in each room, with a toilet and kitchen facilities shared by 150 men; these facilities were also not sufficiently sanitised (Lim and Kok 2020). It was also common practice for two men to 'rotate' on one bed, with the day-shift worker able to sleep on the bed when the night-shift worker is at work, and vice versa (Yea 2020). As I will discuss later in this chapter, these worker dormitory infections represent a significant policy blind-spot that had arisen in shortcomings or deficiencies in analytical capacity.

The Covid-19 pandemic has also given rise to significant socio-economic disruption in Singapore. More than just a healthcare crisis, the economic spill-over effects of the Covid-19 pandemic are expected to cause an economic crisis, not only in Singapore but all over the world. On 14 July 2020, Singapore entered technical recession, with its economy contracting by 41.2% in the second quarter on the back of weak external demand and decreased domestic economic activity due to the circuit breaker (Tang 2020).

The Covid-19 pandemic is expected to cause the worst recession that Singapore has ever experienced. Hence unlike the SARS crisis, Singapore's response to the Covid-19 pandemic necessarily involved a larger gamut of policy tools that targets a broader spectrum of society. These range from economic stimulus packages to strict social distancing rules and new healthcare system procedures. I will now discuss these various policy initiatives in the next section on Singapore's response to the Covid-19 pandemic.

SINGAPORE'S RESPONSE

Like the SARS crisis, the policy initiatives and measures that were implemented during the Covid-19 pandemic can be categorised as:

Community Measures
Healthcare System Measures
International Measures

On 22 January 2020, a Multi-Ministry Taskforce on Covid-19 was established to lead and direct Singapore's response to the Covid-19 pandemic. Co-chaired by Minister for Health Gan Kim Yong and Minister for National Development Lawrence Wong, the Taskforce includes ministers from the various relevant ministries that are expected to be involved in Singapore's Covid-19 response. These are listed in Table 4.1.

The composition of the Multi-Ministry Taskforce also reflects the diverse areas of Singaporean society which have been impacted by the Covid-19 pandemic. Whether in terms of hospital resources (healthcare), disruptions to schools (education) and food supply chains (trade and industry) or even heightened social tensions amidst the circuit breaker (social and family development), the impacts of Covid-19 on Singapore were large and diverse, prompting a multi-pronged approach involving a range of different ministries and ministers.

Community Measures

Unlike the SARS crisis, Covid-19 was not a nosocomial infection. Rather, a large proportion of Covid-19 infections occurred within the broader community. The community measures implemented during the Covid-19 crisis were therefore much more extensive, as compared to those that were implemented during the SARS crisis. Singapore's community measures for managing the Covid-19 pandemic can therefore be further delineated into three distinct categories:

- Safe distancing measures
- Mandated wearing of face masks
- Financial support

Table 4.1   Multi-Ministry Taskforce on Covid-19 (Ministry of Health 2020b)

Role	Member	Ministry/Agency
Co-Chairs	Mr Gan Kim Yong Minister for Health	Ministry of Health
	Mr Lawrence Wong Minister for National Development	Ministry of National Development
Advisor	Mr Heng Swee Keat Deputy Prime Minister	
Members	Mr S Iswaran Minister for Communications and Information	Ministry of Communications and Information
	Mr Chan Chun Sing Minister for Trade and Industry	Ministry of Trade and Industry
	Mr Masagos Zulkifli Minister for the Environment and Water Resources	Ministry of the Environment and Water Resources
	Mr Ng Chee Meng Minister, Prime Minister's Office Secretary-General of National Trades Union Congress	National Trades Union Congress
	Mr Ong Ye Kung Minister for Education	Ministry of Education
	Mrs Josephine Teo Minister for Manpower	Ministry of Manpower
	Mr Desmond Lee Minister for Social and Family Development	Ministry of Social and Family Development
	Dr Janil Puthucheary Senior Minister of State	Ministry of Transport

Safe Distancing

The Covid-19 virus is mainly spread through air-borne droplets that are released when an infected individual sneezes or coughs in public. An infection can occur when a sufficient amount of these droplets is breathed in by a passer-by or close contact. Aside from airborne droplets, the Covid-19 virus can also be spread through contact with contaminated surfaces. Such surfaces could have been contaminated with the afore-mentioned airborne droplets land on these surfaces, or when an infected person touches these surfaces after having sneezed or coughed into his or her hand.

Given this nature of Covid-19's transmission mechanism, Singapore's community measures were therefore strongly centred on social distancing, also known as 'safe distancing' in the city-state. This began on 7 February 2020, with the raising of the DORSCON level from yellow to orange giving rise to the first set of community measures. Specifically, organisers of large-scale public events were advised to defer these events while schools were asked to suspend after-school and external activities. Workplaces were also advised to carry out temperature scanning.

The rapid rise of local Covid-19 cases and clusters would prompt the government to introduce its 'safe distancing' measures on 13 March 2020, which required the deferment or cancellation of all cultural, sports and entertainment events involving 250 participants or more (Ministry of Health 2020c). This requirement would be expanded to include all events and gatherings (Ministry of Health 2020d). The 13 March 2020 directive also required public venues to impose safe distancing measures, such as ensuring that seats are at least one metre apart in restaurants, limiting the number of patrons that can enter entertainment venues, tourist attractions and sports facilities and ensuring that these patrons keep a one metre distance from each other.

On 24 March 2020, the government announced the closure of all bars and entertainment venues, suspension of all religious and worship activities, and the deferment or cancellation of all events and mass gatherings, while other public venues such as malls and public attractions were required to reduce crowd density to no more than one person per 16 square metres of usable space, with museum group tours and mall atrium sales cancelled as well (Ministry of Health 2020e). At the same time, the Multi-Ministry Taskforce also announced stricter measures to limit gatherings outside of work and school to no more than 10 persons.

It was however on 3 April 2020 that Singapore announced its most stringent set of safe distancing rules yet: a 'circuit breaker' that involved the shutting down of all schools and non-essential workplaces. Under the circuit breaker, schools shifted to home-based learning while work was carried out through telecommuting from home. Additionally, the circuit breaker mandated the closure of non-essential retail stores, while restaurants and other food outlets were only allowed to offer takeaway or delivery services. Supermarkets and pharmacies were allowed to resume business, albeit under strict safe distancing guidelines.

Initially planned for a month, the circuit breaker would come to be extended for another month. The circuit breaker was eventually lifted on 1 June 2020 under a phased reopening of Singapore's socio-economic activities.

While Phase 1 allowed for the reopening of schools and workplaces, it was only in Phase 2 that retail stores and food and beverage outlets were allowed to resume operations, albeit under safe distancing measures. Social interactions involving up to 5 people were also allowed. As of writing, Singapore is still operating under Phase 2 conditions. Phase 3 reopening is expected to return Singapore to normal conditions, although this is expected to only take place upon the development of an effective Covid-19 vaccine or treatment.

Face Masks

Aside from social distancing, another key community measure involved the distribution and mandated wearing of face masks in public. In an experiment conducted by the Agency for Science, Technology and Research (A*STAR) and the Singapore General Hospital, scientists found that a properly-worn mask can significantly reduce the spread of droplets from an infected person (Government of Singapore 2020).

While this importance of face masks is evident on hindsight, it was not always the case during the crisis. The WHO only recognised the importance of mandating all individuals to wear a face mask in public in early April 2020, with the consequence being that countries that complied with WHO guidelines and regulations, such as Singapore, faced a similar lag-time in implementing mandatory mask-wearing in public.

Prior to 15 April, the government had maintained its position that individuals should only wear a mask if they are unwell (Zhang 2020). It was only on 3 April 2020 that Prime Minister Lee would announce during a national address that the government would no longer be discouraging people from wearing masks in public; this was on the back of an extensive review of the medical literature by the MOH that was conducted in March (Zhang 2020). This is particularly in light of emerging evidence from the WHO and the U.S. Center for Disease Control and Protection that the virus could be spread by persons who did not display the typical symptoms of Covid-19 infection.

In recognition of the emerging scientific consensus on mask-wearing as well as the WHO's change in stance on mask-wearing, the government updated its mask guidelines to encourage the wearing of masks in public spaces, eventually making it mandatory on 15 April 2020 for individuals to wear a mask whenever they leave their homes or vehicles (Ministry of Health 2020a). Barring several exceptions (such as during strenuous exercise or when travelling in a vehicle with fellow household members), anyone caught outside without a mask would face an initial fine of SG$300, and a fine of SG$1000 for subsequent offences (Yong 2020b).

Budgets

Aside from efforts to reduce social interaction and close contact among individuals, a third set of community measures involved the disbursement of financial resources to mitigate the economic impacts of the pandemic for individuals, households and businesses. This was effected through the unveiling of four budgets in quick succession, an event that was unprecedented in Singapore's independent history.

The first budget was unveiled on 18 February 2020. Known as the "Unity Budget", this first budget drew on SG$6.4 billion to fund the government's efforts to address the impacts of the Covid-19 pandemic. Covid-19-related measures included a SG$1.6 billion Care and Support Scheme that would fund a one-time pay-out of between SG$100 and SG$300 to Singaporeans aged 21 and above, a SG$1.3 billion Job Support Scheme that would pay for 8% of the wages of local workers, as well as various tax rebates for firms in the aviation, hospitality and MICE (meetings, incentives, conventions and exhibitions) sectors that had been hit hard by the Covid-19 crisis.

The budget also included a whole slew of other measures, top-ups and special transfers aimed at stimulating Singapore's economy in what was increasingly recognised as a difficult year ahead. The Unity Budget would be swiftly followed by the announcement of a SG$55 billion "Resilience Budget" on 26 March 2020. Amounting to 11% of Singapore's GDP, the Resilience Budget further enhanced the Jobs Support Scheme by co-funding 25% of the wages of all local workers (raised from the previous level of 8%), with sectors that have been harder hit by the pandemic receiving higher levels of wage co-funding, such as the food services sector (50% wage support) and the aviation and tourism sectors (75% wage support).

The Care and Support Scheme was also significantly expanded, with cash pay-outs to all adult Singaporeans tripled and the introduction of an additional SG$300 pay-out for all parents. Other measures that were introduced include a SG$1.2 billion Self-Employed Person Income Relief Scheme that paid out a monthly case assistance of SG$1000 to self-employed persons, a Temporary Relief Fund that provided financial assistance to the needy, a freeze on all government fees and charges for a year, an automatic 3-month deferment of income tax payments for companies and self-employed persons, as well as a range of property tax rebates and write-offs for businesses that have been especially hard hit by the pandemic.

To address the disruptions that were expected to emerge with the circuit breaker, a SG$5.1 billion "Solidarity Budget" was unveiled on 6 April 2020. The budget further expanded the Care and Support Scheme by providing an additional SG$300 cash pay-out to all adult Singaporeans, with the first tranche of Care and Support Scheme pay-outs brought forward to April 2020 while all other payments that were announced in the Resilience Budget were similarly brought forward to June 2020. The Jobs Support Scheme was similarly expanded, with the government now co-funding 75% of workers' wages across all sectors.

Lastly, a SG$33 billion "Fortitude Budget" was introduced on 26 May 2020 to help businesses and workers tide through the Covid-19 crisis and its deleterious impacts on the economy. The Fortitude Budget included enhancements and extensions to the Job Support Scheme, a SG$2 billion SGUnited Jobs and Skills Package to create 40,000 jobs, 25,000 trainee-ships and 30,000 skills training opportunities, as well as a SG$13 billion contingent sum that could be used to respond to any potential uncertainties that may arise from the pandemic, along with other measures (Lim 2020).

Taken together, the four budgets mobilised close to SG$100 billion to address the Covid-19 crisis, with SG$52 billion drawn from past reserves (Chew 2020, Lim 2020). As I will discuss later in this chapter, Singapore's ability to draw on such large amounts of financial resources to address the Covid-19 crisis reflects its extensive material capacity.

Healthcare System Measures

While Singapore's community measures played an important role in limiting community transmission of the Covid-19 virus by minimising social interactions and contact, its healthcare system measures have been equally, if not more, important in testing, detecting and treating Covid-19 cases.

This began on 23 January 2020, when Singapore's first confirmed Covid-19 case, a 66-year-old Chinese man from Wuhan, was admitted into the Singapore General Hospital's (SGH) isolation ward, with contact tracing initiated immediately. SGH, along with other hospitals, would quickly find their isolation wards and intensive care units (ICUs) filled up as confirmed Covid-19 cases rose rapidly over the subsequent few months. This necessitated the mobilisation of other facilities to house some of the Covid-19 patients.

To this end, the MOH put in place a 'comprehensive medical strategy' that involved a set of 'tiered medical facilities'. Under this strategy, patients who exhibited severe symptoms admitted into the various hospitals' ICUs while those with mild or no symptoms were cared for at Community Care Facilities (CCFs); patients who were recovering were also often transferred to CCFs from the hospitals (Ministry of Health 2020f). The CCFs were established in response to the rising rates of infection that threatened to overwhelm Singapore's healthcare system. These facilities include holiday chalets such as D'Resort in Pasir Ris as well as convention halls that were repurposed to become CCFs, such as Singapore Expo and the Changi Exhibition Centre.

Hence while the NCID and isolation facilities that were established post-SARS reflect the presence of excess capacity, the onset of crisis often requires the optimisation of these resources and capacities in order to preserve healthcare capacity during the crisis. This necessary transition between 'slack' and 'optimisation' in policy capacity will be discussed in the following chapter. The tiered medical facilities that were set up during the Covid-19 outbreak therefore represent a crucial set of healthcare system measures that prevented Singapore's hospitals from becoming overwhelmed by the large number of infections.

Within these tiered medical facilities, healthcare processes and procedures were quickly introduced with the onset of Covid-19. These processes and procedures are broadly similar to those that were introduced during SARS, such as the compulsory use of PPEs by healthcare workers and medical personnel, extensive screening and contact tracing processes at entry points to hospitals and other medical facilities, limitations to the number of visitors to these facilities as well as the deferment of non-essential medical procedures, and perhaps most importantly, the reactivation of a network of Public Healthcare Preparedness Clinics (PHPCs).

Comprising 900 primary care clinics and last activated during the 2009 H1N1 influenza pandemic, the PHPCs were provided with the necessary resources, guidance and PPEs to provide subsidised consultation, treatment, investigations and medications for all Singapore citizens and permanent residents diagnosed with respiratory illnesses (Today Online

2020). This contributed to a greater willingness among the public to seek medical attention for respiratory illnesses, in the process facilitating early detection of Covid-19 infections and reducing community transmission.

Aside from healthcare procedures and facilities, another key set of healthcare system measures include the development and use of Covid-19 test-kits. Firstly, ASTAR and Tan Tock Seng Hospital co-developed the 'Fortitude' swab test kit that would play a crucial role in broader Covid-19 testing across Singapore. While initially used by hospitals, the use of these test kits were subsequently extended to 20 polyclinics and selected general practitioner (GP) clinics, with samples collected processed at the NCID's National Public Health Laboratory as well as private laboratories such as ParkwayHealth Laboratory (Teo 2020a).

This was followed by the development of the world's first serological test by Duke-NUS Medical School, which played a key role in identifying the linkage between two infection clusters (CNA 2020a). Such serological tests that allow researchers to detect antibodies that are developed in an infected person have subsequently been used to assess the extent of community transmission in Singapore. The Duke-NUS Medical School would also subsequently develop a rapid test kit that can detect the presence of Covid-19 antibodies in a person within a few hours (Goh 2020).

A similar emphasis on speed was taken by Singapore-based medical technology firm Biolidics Limited, which developed a test kit that can test for Covid-19 infection in a person within 10 minutes (Kamil 2020). In sum, test kits and testing capabilities represent an important component of Singapore's healthcare response to the Covid-19 pandemic, with rapid test kits contributing to its ability to quickly identify infected persons as well as expedite its contact tracing processes.

While highly effective, these healthcare measures are only focused on detecting and treating Covid-19 cases within Singapore's broader population. It should be noted that even the most efficient or well-developed healthcare system can be overwhelmed by high levels of infection. Given Singapore's position as a global business and tourism hub, large numbers of 'imported' Covid-19 cases could easily enter Singapore and overwhelm its healthcare system.

It was therefore crucial that measures were put in place to limit the importation of Covid-19 cases, in order to preserve healthcare system capacity and functionality. I will now discuss these 'international measures' that were implemented to minimise and limit the potential inflow of Covid-19 cases from overseas.

International Measures

Singapore's first set of international measures were implemented on 2 January 2020, when the MOH began temperature screening for inbound travellers from Wuhan. These temperature screening measures would subsequently be expanded to all incoming travellers from China on 22 January, while anyone with pneumonia and travel history to China within 14 days were required to be isolated. The introduction of these expanded measures coincided with the formation of the Multi-Ministry Task Force. These temperature screening measures can therefore be thought of as an 'automatic' mechanism that is set off with the onset of an emerging epidemic or pandemic in the region, since the Task Force was only established after these measures had already been initiated.

Temperature screening measures would be significantly expanded with the identification of Singapore's first Covid-19 case, with temperature screening implemented at all sea and land checkpoints for all travellers on 23 January 2020. Travel curbs were subsequently introduced on 28 January. Under these travel curbs, visitors with recent travel history to Hubei or with passports issued in Hubei were not allowed to enter or transit in Singapore. These travel curbs were subsequently expanded to on 1 February 2020 to include all visitors of any nationality with recent travel history to Mainland China.

Singapore residents and employment pass-holders returning from China were also required to go on a 14-day stay home notice from 17 February. As Covid-19 infections soared across the world, Singapore announced on 3 March that travellers from Iran, Northern Italy and South Korea would not be allowed to transit or enter Singapore. From 15 March 2020, travellers with recent travel history to ASEAN countries, Japan, Switzerland and the United Kingdom were also issued with a 14-day stay home notice when they entered Singapore. During this period, Singaporean residents were also advised to defer all travel abroad, while all short-term employment pass holders were barred from entering or transiting in Singapore on 22 March 2020.

More stay home notices were subsequently issued, with Singapore residents and pass holders returning from the US and UK required to serve a 14-day stay home notice at dedicated facilities. These facilities largely comprised hotels, many of which were tasked to house returning Singapore residents and pass holders who were required to go on stay home notices. This would serve to prevent these returning individuals from potentially spreading the coronavirus to their family or household members. The commencement of the circuit breaker on 7 April would lead to a complete halt to all travel and transit into Singapore, with the exception of delivery drivers and certain essential services personnel who were allowed to enter Singapore from Malaysia via the Causeway that connects the two countries by land. These broad travel restrictions would be loosened with the end of the circuit breaker. As of writing, the government has allowed travellers from certain countries to transit in its airport, while plans are also afoot to allow cross-border travel between Singapore and Malaysia.

POLICY CAPACITY IN SINGAPORE'S COVID-19 RESPONSES

Singapore's response to the Covid-19 pandemic has involved policy capacity in two key ways. First, it drew upon existing capacities that were established post-SARS. Second, new capacities were created to address the rapidly-worsening Covid-19 pandemic. While some of these capacities were developed through the adaptation or modification of existing capacities, others were entirely new.

In the rest of this chapter, I will discuss the policy capacities that were mobilised and created in Singapore's response to the Covid-19 pandemic. I will also discuss the capacity deficiencies and shortcomings that may have prevented policymakers from preventing the emergence of large infection clusters in Singapore's migrant worker dormitories.

Operational Capacity

At the heart of Singapore's operational capacity is its excellent health-care system. Ranked among the top in the world but taking up relatively low levels of state expenditures, Singapore's healthcare system has been described as "high quality, low cost" (Haseltine 2013). Of particular importance is the availability of hospital beds and resources for treating infected patients. In the early phases of both the SARS and Covid-19 outbreaks, designated hospitals were tasked with receiving and treating infected patients, with the Tan Tock Seng Hospital designated as the 'SARS hospital' while the National Centre for Infectious Diseases (NCID) played a similar role for Covid-19 (Tan 2003).

Completed in May 2019, the NCID is a 330-bed purpose-built medical facility that is "designed to manage an outbreak on the scale of SARS" (Kurohi 2019). The NCID building includes isolation units, in-house laboratories and research units, high-efficiency particular air filters, as well as technological features such as real-time locational contact tracing through electronic tags that are issued to all staff, patients and visitors (Co 2019). Prior to the Covid-19 outbreak, the NCID was mainly involved in detecting and treating major food poisoning cases, and conducting research on infectious diseases (Kurohi 2019).

As I will discuss in the next chapter, the NCID can be thought of as a form of excess capacity that could be tapped on during the outbreak of an infectious disease, but which would otherwise be left to focus on research activities rather than active clinical work. However, even such excess capacity would not be enough, with the rapid increase in Covid-19 cases requiring the government to tap into other hospital and medical facilities for the isolation and treatment of infected patients.

In a bid to preserve hospital capacity, the Ministry of Health announced on 23 March 2020 that Covid-19 patients who are clinically well but continue to test positive for the virus would be transferred to private hospitals such as Concord International Hospital, Mount Elizabeth Hospital and a community isolation facility that was set up at a holiday resort facility in Eastern Singapore (Chong 2020a; CNA 2020b). The Singapore Expo, an exhibition and convention centre in Eastern Singapore, was subsequently converted into a second community isolation facility for Covid-19 patients who are recovering or exhibit mild symptoms (Tee 2020).

A rapid rise in infection rates among Singapore's migrant workers also prompted the government to rehouse many of its healthy migrant workers in other facilities, such as schools, military camps, university student accommodations, and vacant public housing projects, so as to prevent further spread of the virus among migrant workers (Phua and Ang 2020). As I will discuss below, many of these migrant workers were living in highly cramped and often-unsanitary conditions.

As I discuss below, the availability of physical infrastructure is crucial to ensuring operational capacity. While its healthcare infrastructure such as hospitals and clinics has allowed Singapore to house and treat infected persons, the availability of other physical infrastructure that can easily be converted into patient-care and isolation facilities, such as hotels, military barracks, and convention centres, have also contributed immensely to its ability to maintain operational capacity in the face of rising infection rates. Such infrastructure can therefore be thought of as a form of excess capacity, that though not purpose-built for dealing with a pandemic, can nonetheless be mobilised during such a crisis.

Aside from hospital and medical facilities, a second source of operational capacity lies in Singapore's ability to conduct extensive contact tracing. In response to questions about the sources of Singapore's success in managing Covid-19, Prime Minister Lee noted that: "As the cases started to come in, we were able to identify them, because we said treatment and testing for COVID-19 will be free. We were able also to contact trace and find the contacts of the people who had come in and isolate the contacts, so that we slow down the spread within the population" (Lee 2020).

Initially drawn from the Ministry of Health and subsequently incorporating personnel from the Singapore Police Force and the Army, contact tracing teams are tasked with identifying the close contacts of infected persons and ensuring that these close contacts are isolated and quarantined to prevent further spread. The contract tracing process begins in the hospital, where a warded patient is asked to construct an 'activity map' that details the activities that he or she has carried out and people that he or she has met over the past two weeks; this is followed by an investigative process whereby contact tracing teams call up all the people that the patient has interacted with, in order to determine whether a person is a close contact and hence at risk of an infection (Khalik 2020). Close contacts who are clinically well are then quarantined for 14 days, while close contacts with coronavirus symptoms are hospitalised.

This ability to conduct extensive contact tracing hinges upon two key capacities. First, it requires personnel who are sufficiently trained to carry out contact tracing. Should infection rates outpace the abilities of contract tracers from the Ministry of Health, relevant personnel from other parts of the public service, such as investigative officers from the police force and military can also be activated. Second, contact tracing requires the presence of established procedures detailing the contract tracing process, such that existing and new contact tracers can quickly take on their roles. In the case of Singapore, these procedures were established in the aftermath of the SARS crisis and encoded in the institutional fabrics of both the Ministry of Health and the NCID.

Another operational capacity that is tangentially related to Singapore's healthcare system and contact tracing efforts is its technological infrastructure. A key example of this is the invention of the Infrared Fever Screening System by the Defence Science and Technology Agency

(DSTA) during the SARS outbreak (Tan et al. 2004). An infrared-based system that allows for fever screening of large groups of people, the Infrared Fever Screening System was deployed at major public buildings and facilities such as the airport during both the SARS outbreak and the Covid-19 pandemic. The DSTA also developed a low-cost diagnostic kit that can detect the presence of the Covid-19 novel coronavirus in individuals in a significantly shorter amount of time (Tan 2020).

More recently, a contact tracing application, the 'TraceTogether app", was developed by the Government Technology Agency (GovTech) and Ministry of Health to assist in its contact tracing efforts. The app identifies people who have been within two metres of coronavirus patients for at least 30 minutes through the use of Bluetooth wireless technology and allows contact tracers to quickly identify other users who have been in close contact with infected persons, rather than relying on individuals' memories (Baharudin 2020a; Government Digital Services 2020). A wearable device was also designed for distribution to individuals who may not have access to smart phones, and hence are not able to use the TraceTogether app (Baharudin 2020b).

It should however be noted that the TraceTogether app was popular with citizens, having been downloaded by only a quarter of the resident population (Chong 2020b). Such reluctance to download the app stemmed in part from limitations in the app that had caused excessive draining of smartphone batteries and in part from privacy concerns (Chong 2020b). GovTech has also adapted the social messaging app Whatsapp to provide citizens with daily updates on Covid-19 cases by developing an artificial intelligence (AI) translation tool and created an app-based reporting tool for monitoring individuals under quarantine (Basu 2020).

Aside from digital technologies, the private technological firm Razer and the DSTA have both been engaged to design produce essential PPEs such as face masks and face shields (CNA 2020c; Koh 2020). These have served to shore up Singapore's supply of masks and PPEs. Like physical infrastructure, the presence of a technological ecosystem comprising technological firms and government technology agencies therefore represents an important facet of Singapore's operational capacities. While these firms and agencies are in ordinary times focused on commercially-viable technologies, they can be mobilised during a pandemic to develop new technologies that can in turn be applied to the government's pandemic response efforts.

Material Capacity

Singapore's ability to develop and mobilise these operational capacities, whether these are healthcare system capabilities or physical and technological infrastructure, fundamentally depended on the availability of material capacity. Three forms of material capacity are especially relevant here. These are financial resources, facilities and technological hardware.

As I have discussed earlier in this chapter, Singapore had over the course of its response to the Covid-19 pandemic introduced four budgets, totalling close to SG $100 billion, with SG $52 billion drawn from its past reserves (Chew 2020). The various features and components of the four budgets have been discussed above, and there is no need to repeat these. It suffices to say, however, that the four budgets aimed to introduce a strong fiscal stimulus to counteract the negative economic impacts of the Covid-19 pandemic as well as to provide for the additional operational capacities that were mobilised during the crisis.

Underpinning this significant financial outlay is Singapore's large national reserves. According to the Ministry of Finance, Singapore's reserves refer to the total assets minus liabilities of the government and its various entities, with total assets comprising physical assets such as land and building and financial assets such as cash, securities and bonds (Ministry of Finance Singapore 2018). Singapore's reserves are managed and invested for returns by its sovereign wealth fund GIC Limited, government-owned investment company Temasek Holdings, and Singapore's central bank, the Monetary Authority of Singapore (MAS).

While the size of Singapore's total reserves are kept secret due to its strategic nature, although estimates by analysts have placed it well above SG $500 billion (Ng and Jaipragas 2019). Current reserves represent the amount of reserve that is accumulated within a term of government, while past reserves consist of the total amount of reserves that have been saved up over past terms of government. While current reserves are used to fund the government's policies and initiatives, the government can also draw from its past reserves during periods of crises, although draw-downs of past reserves require the approval of the elected President.

Singapore's large reserves are therefore an important form of material capacity which allows for the funding of key policy initiatives, particularly during crises. Its past reserves have also been mobilised during the 2009 Global Financial Crisis and during the Covid-19 pandemic, as discussed above. Aside from financial resources, Singapore has also drawn on other forms of material capacity to address the Covid-19 pandemic.

The first of these is its 'national stockpile', which includes more than three months' worth of carbohydrates (such as rice and noodles) and more than two months' worth of proteins and vegetables (Lam 2020). This national stockpile of essential products was initially established to pre-empt disruptions in food supply from Malaysia. In light of heightened demand for masks during the Covid-19 pandemic, the Singapore has also built up a national stockpile of masks and medical supplies (Meah 2020).

Underpinning these stockpiles is the government's ongoing efforts to diversify its supply chains, especially in anticipation of potential disruptions, whether these be due to a pandemic or strategic conflict. This approach is fundamentally driven by Singapore's 'siege mentality' approach to security and diplomacy, as discussed in Chapter 1 (Leifer 2000). In any case, Singapore's national stockpile of food and medical supplies can be seen as an important form of material capacity that can be mobilised during a crisis.

The last form of material capacity that has been particularly relevant in Singapore's Covid-19 response efforts is its urban infrastructure. As I have discussed above, the emergence of large infection clusters in Singapore's migrant worker dormitories had prompted the government to relocated some healthy migrant workers to schools and military barracks that had been repurposed to become temporary worker housing facilities. This served to lower the density of migrant worker dormitories, reducing risks of infection for their residents.

At the same time, exhibition centres such as Singapore Expo and the Changi Exhibition Centre as well as holiday resorts such as D'Resort were also repurposed to become Community Care Facilities (CCFs) to house Covid-19 patients who were clinically well, i.e. exhibiting mild or no symptoms from the virus. Hotels were also mobilised to house returning residents who had to be placed on Stay Home Notice. In sum, urban infrastructure such as hotels, exhibition centres, schools and barracks were rapidly mobilised and repurposed to house Covid-19 patients and individuals on Stay Home Notice.

Whether in the form of financial resources, the national stockpile or urban infrastructure, material capacity represents an important set of resources that can be mobilised during a crisis. Material capacity is particularly crucial for maintaining operational capacity. For instance, financial resources are needed for maintaining existing healthcare system capacity or funding new healthcare initiatives. Similarly, the mobilisation of urban infrastructure to house Covid-19 patents can help conserve healthcare system capacity. Given the role of these material capacities in funding and driving Singapore's Covid-19 response, it is likely that the government will continue to maintain its high levels of material capacity.

However, and as I will discuss in the next chapter, such efforts to maintain a high level of material capacity runs counter to the resource optimisation and efficiency-focus that characterises the dominant NPM approach to public administration. Rather, maintaining high levels of material capacity involves setting aside excess capacity, whether these are financial resources, food or buildings, in preparation for a potential crisis. More importantly, the maintenance of excess capacity can ensure greater systemic robustness during a crisis. Another set of capacities that can contribute to policy robustness is analytical capacity. I will now discuss these.

Analytical Capacity

While the capacities that I have discussed so far have proven crucial in driving Singapore's policy responses during the Covid-19 pandemic, the capacities that it has built up before and in anticipation of the pandemic are equally important. At the heart of such efforts is analytical capacity.

Analytical capacity, particularly in terms of the ability to pre-empt and prepare for a future pandemic draws, significantly on specific and highly technical activities such as strategic foresight and horizon scanning, all of which involve extensive collection and processing of data in order to separate the 'signal' from the 'noise', in the parlance of futurists and foresight specialists. At the heart of such analytical capacities is the government's Centre for Strategic Futures (CSF), a strategic foresight and horizon scanning unit situated within the Prime Minister's Office.

A key aspect of the CSF's role includes "building capacities, mindsets, expertise and tools for strategic anticipation and risk management" (Centre for Strategic Futures 2020). The CSF is therefore tasked with building the tools and capacities for addressing future crises, with pandemics often included as a major high-risk event in the CSF's annual reports (Centre for Strategic Futures 2017).

Aside from pre-empting future pandemics, Singapore's efforts to contain the Covid-19 virus depended heavily on its ability to collect and process large amounts of information, particularly in its contact tracing and quarantine management processes. The role of contact tracing teams as well as the manpower resources that were directed towards contact tracing, both from the MOH and from the military and police force, have been discussed at great length above.

Aside from manpower resources, another important source of analytical capacity are the technological tools that been developed to enhance the Singapore's contact tracing and surveillance abilities. This includes the abovementioned TraceTogether app and the SafeEntry app, a "national digital check-in system" that allows workplaces, malls, restaurants, supermarkets and other public venues to keep track of the individuals who enter their premises, by requiring individuals to 'check-in' to a premise by scanning a QR code (GovTech 2020).

These technological tools can be thought of as an additional means through which the Singaporean government has been able to collect and rapidly process individual locational data, often through automated processes. Such technologically-enabled surveillance tools therefore represent another important form of analytical capacity that has been used, not only in Singapore but in other Asian countries such as South Korea, to keep track of infection rates as well as enforce compliance with quarantine orders.

While these analytical capacities have contributed immensely to Singapore's ability to detect, contain and monitor Covid-19 infections, shortcomings or deficiencies in analytical capacity have also in part driven Singapore's high infection rates, particularly within its migrant worker dormitories.

The emergence of the migrant worker dormitory clusters can be seen as a 'black elephant' event, i.e. an unexpected shock that has arisen from an already-known systemic problem that policymakers and society are unwilling to address (Ho 2008; Centre for Strategic Futures 2017). The cramped and unsanitary conditions of migrant worker dormitories are not new to the public. Much of these had previously been documented published by the media and non-profit organisations such as Transient Workers Count Too (CNA 2018; Transient Workers Count Too 2020).

Yet despite the availability of such information, policymakers were not able to translate this knowledge into 'actionable intelligence' for preventing COVID-19 infections. This inability to translate such information on migrant worker dormitory conditions into healthcare policy implications reflects shortcomings or deficiencies in analytical capacity (Woo 2020). There are several possible reasons for this. First, observers have noted how the government had placed an overly-strong focus on Singaporean citizens and residents in its initial testing and control measures (Nortajuddin 2020). Early and extensive testing of migrant workers residing in these dormitories could have prevented, or at least reduced, these infection clusters.

Second, non-profit and civil society groups who possessed information on the living conditions of these migrant workers were not able to obtain the attention of policymakers. Certainly, much of this can be attributed to the "weak and emasculated" state of Singapore's civil society, exacerbated by a "political acquiescence of the middle class" that had led to state domination of public and societal discourse (Chong 2011). Furthermore, the ability of civil society groups to gain the attention of the government is also unequally distributed across sectors, with areas such as environmental sustainability and women's rights commanding greater policy salience than migrant worker rights (Chua 2000; Chong 2011; Ortmann 2015; Soon and Koh 2017).

Insufficient channels of communication between policymakers and civil society therefore prevented the transmission of important information on migrant worker dormitories onto the policy agenda. Without such information, or the ability to identify the healthcare implications of migrant workers' living conditions, policymakers were effectively blindsided by the large numbers of Covid-19 infections that emerged from migrant worker dormitories.

As I will discuss at the end of this chapter and in the next, certain forms of analytical capacities need to be strengthened, particularly the ability to identify causal linkages across different policy issues and domains, as well as the ability to leverage on the data and information that reside within civil society and to transform this knowledge into actionable intelligence. This latter point—better communication between civil society and the state—also relates to another set of policy capacity, specifically political capacity. I will discuss these next.

Political Capacity

There are two aspects of political capacity that are relevant to the case of Singapore. The first comprises political trust and legitimacy, while the second involves political communications. The two forms of political capacity are interlinked. While the public's willingness to comply with the government's regulations and directives depend on the presence of political trust, effective political communications can serve to build up this trust. Both communications and trust are therefore crucial for ensuring public compliance with policies and regulations, in the process contributing to the successful attainment of policy objectives.

Much has been written about political trust and legitimacy in Singapore. As an archetypal East Asian 'developmental state' that operates on the basis of performance legitimacy, political trust in Singapore is dependent on the government's ability to attain high levels of economic growth and socio-political stability (Huff 1995; Perry et al. 1997; Liow 2011; Woo 2018). Singapore's success in managing past crises and pandemics, such as the SARS crisis and the 2007 Global Financial Crisis, would have likely contributed to the government's performance legitimacy.

Some of this can also be attributed to the Singaporean state's 'semiauthoritarian' approach to governance and its low tolerance for dissent (George 2007; Rodan 2008; Tan 2012, 2016), although the People's Action Party's (PAP) ability to consistently win all General Elections since Singapore's independence allude to a relatively high level of political trust from the general population. Certainly, the recent 2020 General Elections suggest some level of decline in this trust and the government's performance legitimacy, with the PAP experiencing an 8% decline in vote-share and the lost off a GRC to the opposition Workers' Party.

While some observers had attributed this decline in vote-share to citizens' unhappiness with the government's handling of the Covid-19 pandemic (BBC 2020; Li 2020), others have pointed to public unhappiness over the government's decision to hold an election during the pandemic in the first place (Koh 2020). The PAP's own assessment was that voters in their 40s and 50s had voted against it due to the economic hardships that had arisen from the pandemic, while its online campaign was not able to connect well with younger voters (Lai 2020). This was despite expectations, based on historical precedence, that the PAP would do well during the elections due to a 'flight to safety' mentality among voters (Li 2020).

However, one should also not read too much into the elections results. The PAP's ability to secure a 61.2% vote-share suggests broad general support from the population, while continued public compliance with safe distancing rules and measures point to a certain level of trust in the government's ability to manage the Covid-19 pandemic.

Aside from issues of trust and legitimacy, political communications have also played a key role in ensuring public compliance. Singapore's efforts to communicate its policies to the general public, particularly during the early phases of the Covid-19 pandemic, has received much favourable attention. Much of this has been attributed to the government's clear and concise policy directions and advice that were delivered through traditional and social media on a near-daily basis (Hsu and Tan 2020; Sagar 2020).

This emphasis on trust and transparency in political communications was also evident during the SARS crisis, with the government granting World Health Organisation (WHO) officials full access to its information and all data and information presented in a daily conference chaired by the Director of Medical Services and attended by key public officials and WHO observers (Centre for Strategic Futures 2017, p. 14). This practice of daily information sharing has been extended to the Covid-19 crisis, with the Multi-Ministry Taskforce on Covid-19 sharing updates and information with the public through frequent press conferences.

Yet despite these efforts, insufficient communications between the government and dormitory operators as well as employers of construction workers may have led to the commingling of workers from different dormitories at worksites and in social settings. This was revealed in a ministerial statement by Manpower Minister Josephine Teo on 4 May 2020, with infected workers from different dormitories found to be linked through common worksites (Teo 2020b). While the first dormitory cluster was identified on 30 March 2020, the practice of allowing workers from different dormitories to work on common worksites continued well into early May.

Dormitory workers and construction sector employers were therefore not sufficiently cognizant of the infection risks that can emerge when workers from different dormitories go to work at common worksites and return to their individual dormitories at the end of the workday. This suggests some limitations in Singapore's political communications, particularly in terms of the government's ability to effectively communicate its policy stance and regulations to dormitory operators and construction sector employers.

Conclusion

As this chapter has shown, Singapore's ability to respond quickly to the Covid-19 pandemic and minimise Covid-19-related fatalities is fundamentally driven by the presence of key policy capacities that allowed it to identify and isolate potential Covid-19 cases, maintain healthcare system capacity and functionality despite high infection rates, provide the necessary financial and material resources to support its Covid-19 response, and ensure public compliance with its policy initiatives and regulations, among others.

At the same time, its high rate of infection, much of it driven by large infection clusters within its migrant worker dormitories, are also attributable to deficiencies in certain analytical capacities, with the result being insufficient understanding of the infection risks that resided within these cramped and densely-populated migrant worker dormitories. This suggests a need to strengthen those aspects of analytical capacity that can enhance policymakers' understanding of migrant worker dormitory conditions as well as those that can help policymakers develop a keener understanding of the causal linkages that may exist between different policy issues and domains—in this case, linkages between manpower policy and healthcare policy.

Policy capacity is therefore a useful frame of analysis that can help policymakers and researchers to identify the strengths and limitations that may exist within their policy systems. As Singapore's experience with Covid-19 has shown, a deep pool of excess policy capacity is necessary for rapid response to crises, even if this runs counter to NPM expectations of resource optimisation and efficiency. Conversely, the framing of policy limitations in terms of capacity deficiencies can help policymakers identify the specific capacities that may need to be built up, in order that future crisis response efforts are improved and enhanced. I will discuss these at greater length in the next chapter.

References

Baharudin, H. (2020a). Coronavirus: S'pore Government to Make Its Contact-Tracing App Freely Available to Developers Worldwide [online]. *The Straits Times*. Available from: https://www.straitstimes.com/singapore/corona virus-spore-government-to-make-its-contact-tracing-app-freely-available-to. Accessed 9 April 2020.

Baharudin, H. (2020b). Wearable Device for Covid-19 Contact Tracing to Be Rolled Out Soon, May Be Issued to Everyone in Singapore [online]. *The Straits Times*. Available from: https://www.straitstimes.com/politics/parlia ment-wearable-device-for-contact-tracing-set-to-be-issued-tracetogether-does-not-work. Accessed 15 June 2020.

Basu, M. (2020). *Exclusive: How Singapore Sends Daily Whatsapp Updates on Coronavirus| GovInsider* [online]. GovInsider. Available from: https://govins ider.asia/innovation/singapore-coronavirus-whatsapp-covid19-open-govern ment-products-govtech/. Accessed 31 March 2020.

BBC. (2020, July 10). *Singapore Ruling Party Wins Poll But Support Falls*. BBC News..

Centre for Strategic Futures. (2017). *Foresight*. Singapore: Prime Minister's Office Singapore.

Centre for Strategic Futures. (2020). *Who We Are* [online]. Prime Minister's Office Singapore. Available from: https://www.csf.gov.sg/who-we-are/. Accessed 9 April 2020.

Chew, H. M. (2020). *Parliament Passes Fortitude Budget, 4th Package of COVID-19 Relief Measures This Year* [online]. CNA. Available from: https://www.channelnewsasia.com/news/singapore/fortitude-budget-covid-19-parliament-passes-heng-swee-keat-12808172. Accessed 19 July 2020.

Chong, C. (2020a). Patients Who Are Well But Still Testing Positive for Covid-19 to Be Moved to Community Isolation Facility to Preserve Hospital Capacity [online]. *The Straits Times*. Available from: https://www.straitstimes.com/singapore/patients-who-are-well-but-still-testing-positive-for-covid-19-to-be-moved-to-community. Accessed 1 April 2020.

Chong, C. (2020b). About 1 Million People Have Downloaded TraceTogether App, But More Need to do so for It to Be Effective: Lawrence Wong [online]. *The Straits Times*. Available from: https://www.straitstimes.com/singapore/about-one-million-people-have-downloaded-the-tracetogether-app-but-more-need-to-do-so-for. Accessed 8 June 2020.

Chong, T. (2011). Civil Society in Singapore: Popular Discourses and Concepts. *Sojourn: Journal of Social Issues in Southeast Asia, 20*(2), 273–301.

Chua, B. H. (2000). The Relative Autonomies of State and Civil Society in Singapore. In G. Koh & G. L. Ooi (Eds.), *State-Society Relations in Singapore* (pp. 62–76). Singapore: Institute of Policy Studies.

CNA. (2018). *Construction Company Fined for Housing Foreign Workers in Cramped, Filthy Conditions* [online]. CNA. Available from: https://www.channelnewsasia.com/news/singapore/construction-company-keong-hong-fined-foreign-workers-housing-10285764. Accessed 26 May 2020.

CNA. (2020a). *Duke-NUS Used COVID-19 Antibody Tests to Establish Link Between Church Clusters in a World-First* [online]. CNA. Available from: https://www.channelnewsasia.com/news/singapore/covid19-coronavirus-duke-nus-antibody-tests-12469184. Accessed 27 May 2020.

CNA. (2020b). *COVID-19 Patients Who Are 'Well and Stable' to Be Transferred to Selected Private Hospitals: MOH* [online]. CNA. Available from: https://www.channelnewsasia.com/news/singapore/covid-19-patients-transferred-private-hospitals-capacity-12568750. Accessed 1 April 2020.

CNA. (2020c). *Razer's Face Mask Manufacturing Line Begins Production, Able to Produce 5 Million Masks a Month* [online]. CNA. Available from: https://www.channelnewsasia.com/news/singapore/razer-face-mask-manufacturing-covid-19-5-million-12673442. Accessed 14 June 2020.

Co, C. (2019). *New Infectious Diseases Centre to Have Real-Time Location Tracking* [online]. CNA. Available from: https://www.channelnewsasia.com/news/singapore/ncid-national-centre-for-infectious-diseases-singapore-11882690. Accessed 1 April 2020.

George, C. (2007). Consolidating Authoritarian Rule: Calibrated Coercion in Singapore. *The Pacific Review, 20*(2), 127–145.

Goh, T. (2020). Duke-NUS Scientists Develop Speedy Test for Antibodies That Can Neutralise Coronavirus [online]. *The Straits Times*. Available from: https://www.straitstimes.com/singapore/health/duke-nus-scientists-develop-speedy-test-for-antibodies-that-can-neutralise. Accessed 1 June 2020.

Government Digital Services. (2020). *TraceTogether* [online]. Available from: https://www.tracetogether.gov.sg/. Accessed 9 April 2020.

Government of Singapore. (2020). *The Science Behind Why Masks Help Prevent COVID-19 Spread* [online]. Available from: http://www.gov.sg/article/the-science-behind-why-masks-help-prevent-covid-19-spread. Accessed 17 May 2020.

GovTech. (2020). *SafeEntry—National Digital Check-in System* [online]. Available from: https://safeentry.gov.sg/. Accessed 25 May 2020.

Haseltine, W. A. (2013). *Affordable Excellence: The Singapore Healthcare Story: How to Create and Manage Sustainable Healthcare Systems*. Washington, DC: Brookings Institution Press.

Ho, P. (2008). *Governing at the Leading Edge: Black Swans, Wild Cards, and Wicked Problems*. Singapore: Institute of Southeast Asian Studies.

Hsu, L. Y., & Tan, M.-H. (2020). *What Singapore Can Teach the U.S. About Responding to Covid-19*. STAT.

Huff, W. G. (1995). The Developmental State, Government, and Singapore's Economic Development Since 1960. *World Development, 23*(8), 1421–1438.

Kamil, A. (2020). Local Firm Develops Rapid Test Kit That Can Detect Covid-19 in Less Than 10 Minutes [online]. *TODAYonline*. Available from: https://www.todayonline.com/singapore/local-firm-develops-rapid-test-kit-can-detect-covid-19-less-10-minutes. Accessed 1 June 2020.

Khalik, S. (2020). Coronavirus: How Contact Tracers Track Down the People at Risk of Infection [online]. *The Straits Times*. Available from: https://www.straitstimes.com/singapore/health/how-contact-tracers-track-down-the-people-at-risk-of-infection. Accessed 31 March 2020.

Koh, F. (2020). DSTA Face Shield to Protect Front-Line Workers in Coron-avirus Fight [online]. *The Straits Times*. Available from: https://www.strait stimes.com/singapore/dsta-face-shield-to-protect-front-line-workers-in-virus-fight. Accessed 14 June 2020.

Koh, F. (2020). Singapore GE: Opposition Parties Criticise Timing of Bound-aries Report, Say Election Should Not Be Held During Covid-19 Pandemic [online]. *The Straits Times*. Available from: https://www.straitstimes.com/politics/singapore-ge-opposition-parties-criticise-timing-of-boundaries-rep ort-say-election-should. Accessed 24 July 2020.

Kurohi, R. (2019, January 17). Centre to Boost Infectious Disease Management. *The Straits Times*, p. B3.

Lai, L. (2020). GE2020 Results a 'Clear Mandate' Although 61.2 Per cent Vote Share Lower Than 65 Per cent PAP Hoped for: Lawrence Wong, Politics News & Top Stories [online]. *The Straits Times*. Available from: https://www.straitstimes.com/politics/singapore-ge2020-results-a-clear-mandate-tho ugh-61-2-per-cent-vote-share-was-lower-than-65. Accessed 24 July 2020.

Lam, L. (2020). *Singapore Has Months' Worth of Stockpiles, Planned for Disruption of Supplies from Malaysia for Years: Chan Chun Sing* [online]. CNA. Available from: https://www.channelnewsasia.com/news/singapore/coronavirus-covid-19-chan-chun-sing-food-supply-12545326. Accessed 20 July 2020.

Lee, H. L. (2020). *PM Lee Hsien Loong's Interview with CNN* [online]. Prime Minister's Office Singapore. Available from: http://www.pmo.gov.sg/New sroom/PM-interview-with-CNN. Accessed 31 March 2020.

Leifer, M. (2000). *Singapore's Foreign Policy: Coping with Vulnerability*. London: Routledge.

Li, N. (2020). A *'New Mandate' for Singapore's Government?* [online]. Available from: https://thediplomat.com/2020/07/a-new-mandate-for-sin gapores-government/. Accessed 24 July 2020.

Lim, K., & Kok, X. (2020). Singapore's Cramped Migrant Worker Dorms a 'Perfect Storm' for Rising Coronavirus Infections [online]. *South China Morning Post*. Available from: https://www.scmp.com/week-asia/health-env ironment/article/3078684/singapores-cramped-migrant-worker-dorms-per fect-storm. Accessed 6 August 2020.

Lim, Y. L. (2020). $33b Set Aside in Fortitude Budget, Bringing Singapore's Covid-19 War Chest to Nearly $100 Billion [online]. *The Straits Times*. Available from: https://www.straitstimes.com/politics/parliament-33-billion-set-aside-in-fortitude-budget-bringing-covid-19-war-chest-to-nearly. Accessed 27 May 2020.

Liow, E. D. (2011). The Neoliberal-Developmental State: Singapore as Case Study. *Critical Sociology*. https://doi.org/10.1177/0896920511419900.

Meah, N. (2020). Singapore Is Building Up Mask Stockpile, But People Should Not Take Availability of Masks for Granted: Chan Chun Sing [online]. *TODAYonline*. Available from: https://www.todayonline.com/singapore/sin gapore-building-mask-stockpile-people-should-not-take-availability-masks-gra nted-chan-chun. Accessed 20 July 2020.

Ministry of Finance Singapore. (2018). *Our Nation's Reserves* [online]. Available from: https://www.mof.gov.sg/policies/our-nation's-reserves/Section-I-What-comprises-the-reserves-and-who-manages-them. Accessed 25 June 2020.

Ministry of Health. (2020a). *Circuit Breaker to Minimise Further Spread of Covid-19* [online]. Available from: https://www.moh.gov.sg/news-highli ghts/details/circuit-breaker-to-minimise-further-spread-of-covid-19. Accessed 16 May 2020.

Ministry of Health. (2020b). *Multi-Ministry Taskforce on Wuhan Coronavirus*.

Ministry of Health. (2020c). *Additional Precautionary Measures to Prevent Further Importation and Spread of Covid-19 Cases* [online]. Ministry of Health Singapore. Available from: https://www.moh.gov.sg/news-highli ghts/details/additional-precautionary-measures-to-prevent-further-import ation-and-spread-of-covid-19-cases. Accessed 18 May 2020.

Ministry of Health. (2020d). *Stricter Safe Distancing Measures to Prevent Further Spread of Covid-19 Cases* [online]. Ministry of Health Singapore. Available from: https://www.moh.gov.sg/news-highlights/details/stricter-safe-distancing-measures-to-prevent-further-spread-of-covid-19-cases. Accessed 18 May 2020.

Ministry of Health. (2020e). *Tighter Measures to Minimise Further Spread of Covid-19* [online]. Ministry of Health Singapore. Available from: https://www.moh.gov.sg/news-highlights/details/tighter-mea sures-to-minimise-further-spread-of-covid-19. Accessed 18 May 2020.

Ministry of Health. (2020f). *Comprehensive Medical Strategy for Covid-19* [online]. Available from: https://www.moh.gov.sg/news-highlights/details/ comprehensive-medical-strategy-for-covid-19. Accessed 28 May 2020.

Ng, J. Y., & Jaipragas, B. (2019). Singapore's Giant Reserves: A Taxing Question for Heng Swee Keat [online]. *South China Morning Post*. Available from: https://www.scmp.com/week-asia/politics/article/2186409/sin gapores-giant-reserves-taxing-question-its-next-prime-minister. Accessed 12 May 2020.

Nortajuddin, A. (2020). *Migrant Worker Cluster: A Singapore Nightmare* [online]. The ASEAN Post. Available from: https://theaseanpost.com/art icle/migrant-worker-cluster-singapore-nightmare. Accessed 22 May 2020.

Ortmann, S. (2015). Political Change and Civil Society Coalitions in Singapore. *Government and Opposition, 50*(1), 119–139.

Perry, M., Kong, L., & Yeoh, B. (1997). *Singapore: A Developmental City State.* Chichester: Wiley.

Phua, R., & Ang, H. M. (2020). '*Dedicated Strategy' to Break COVID-19 Spread in Dormitories, Including Housing Healthy Workers in Army Camps* [online]. CNA. Available from: https://www.channelnewsasia.com/news/singapore/covid-19-foreign-worker-dormitories-range-of-measures-12625624. Accessed 6 May 2020.

Rodan, G. (2008). Singapore "Exceptionalism"? Authoritarian Rule and State Transformation. In J. Wong & E. Friedman (Eds.), *Political Transitions in Dominant Party Systems: Learning to Lose* (pp. 231–251). New York: Routledge.

Sagar, M., 2020. *How Singapore Government's Communication Keeps Nation Moving Forward in Crisis.* OpenGov Asia.

Soon, C., & Koh, G. (Eds.). (2017). *Civil Society and the State in Singapore.* London: World Scientific Europe.

Tan, A. (2020). Coronavirus: Made-in-Singapore Diagnostics Test Implemented in Hospitals Here [online]. *The Straits Times.* Available from: https://www.straitstimes.com/singapore/health/made-in-singapore-diagnostics-test-implemented-in-hospitals-here. Accessed 10 April 2020.

Tan, C. C. (2003). *National Response to SARS.* Singapore.

Tan, K. P. (2012). The Ideology of Pragmatism: Neo-Liberal Globalisation and Political Authoritarianism in Singapore. *Journal of Contemporary Asia, 42*(1), 67–92.

Tan, K. P. (2016). *Governing Global-City Singapore: Legacies and Futures After Lee Kuan Yew.* New York: Routledge.

Tan, M., How, M., Koay, A., & Yap, R. (2020). *4 in S'pore Infected with Wuhan Virus Due to Chinese Tourist Stop in Lavender* [online]. Mothership.sg. Available from: https://mothership.sg/2020/02/wuhan-virus-local-spread/. Accessed 16 May 2020.

Tan, Y. H., Teo, C. W., Ong, E., Tan, B. L., & Soo, M. J. (2004). Development and Deployment of Infrared Fever Screening Systems. *Proceedings of SPIE—The International Society for Optical Engineering.*

Tang, S. K. (2020). *Singapore in Technical Recession After GDP Shrinks 41.2% in Q2 from Preceding Quarter Due to COVID-19* [online]. CNA. Available from: https://www.channelnewsasia.com/news/business/gdp-singapore-technical-recession-contraction-q2-mti-12927168. Accessed 16 July 2020.

Tee, Z. (2020). S'pore Expo 2nd Facility for Community Isolation [online]. *The Straits Times.* Available from: https://www.straitstimes.com/singapore/health/spore-expo-2nd-facility-for-community-isolation. Accessed 8 April 2020.

Teo, J. (2020a). All 20 Polyclinics and Some GPs Can Now Perform Coronavirus Swab Test [online]. *The Straits Times.* Available from: https://www.str

aitstimes.com/singapore/all-19-polyclinics-and-some-gps-can-now-perform-coronavirus-swab-test. Accessed 1 June 2020.

Teo, J. (2020b). *Ministerial Statement by Mrs Josephine Teo, Minister for Manpower* [online]. Ministry of Manpower Singapore. Available from: https://www.mom.gov.sg/newsroom/parliament-questions-and-replies/2020/0504-ministerial-statement-by-mrs-josephine-teo-minister-for-man power-4-may-2020. Accessed 6 August 2020.

Today Online. (2020). Covid-19: MOH Reactivates GPs Network to Limit Community Spread; Subsidies to Be Given for Patients with Respiratory Symptoms [online]. *TODAYonline*. Available from: https://www.todayo nline.com/singapore/moh-reactivates-gps-network-limit-community-spread-subsidies-be-given-patients-respiratory. Accessed 1 June 2020.

Transient Workers Count Too. (2020). *Facts, Research, Analysis*. TWC2.

Woo, J. J. (2018). *The Evolution of the Asian Developmental State: Hong Kong and Singapore*. London: Routledge.

Woo, J. J. (2020). Policy Capacity and Singapore's Response to the COVID-19 Pandemic. *Policy and Society, 0*(0), 1–18.

Yea, S. (2020). This Is Why Singapore's Coronavirus Cases Are Growing: A Look Inside the Dismal Living Conditions of Migrant Workers [online]. *The Conversation*. Available from: http://theconversation.com/this-is-why-sin gapores-coronavirus-cases-are-growing-a-look-inside-the-dismal-living-condit ions-of-migrant-workers-136959. Accessed 6 August 2020.

Yong, M. (2020a). *Timeline: How the COVID-19 Outbreak Has Evolved in Singapore So Far* [online]. CNA. Available from: https://www.channelnewsa sia.com/news/singapore/singapore-covid-19-outbreak-evolved-coronavirus-deaths-timeline-12639444. Accessed 16 May 2020.

Yong, M. (2020b). *COVID-19: What the Law Says About Having to Wear a Mask When Outside Your Home* [online]. CNA. Available from: https://www.channelnewsasia.com/news/singapore/covid-19-sin gapore-masks-going-out-law-12643120. Accessed 20 May 2020.

Zhang, J. (2020). *How S'pore Went from 'Wear a Mask Only If You Are Sick' to 'It Is a Must to Wear Masks' in 3 Months* [online]. Mothership.sg. Available from: https://mothership.sg/2020/04/covid-19-mask-wearing-explainer-sin gapore/. Accessed 20 May 2020.

CHAPTER 5

Conclusion

Abstract In this concluding chapter, I will provide readers with a brief summary of the key arguments and findings that have been presented in the previous chapters. This will allow me to present a broad policy capacity framework that will be useful for policymakers and practitioners who may be interested in building up the necessary capacities for dealing with future pandemics. I will also discuss potential areas for future research conceptualization. This will be useful for readers from research and academia, who may be interested in pursuing further research into policy capacity and crisis management themselves.

Keywords Covid-19 · Policy capacity · Pandemic response · Crisis management

The Covid-19 pandemic has generated massive social, economic and political disruptions across the world. As of writing, there are more than 14.6 million confirmed cases of infection, with reported deaths from the coronavirus exceeding 600,000. The economic impacts of the virus are equally severe. According to the World Bank, the Covid-19 pandemic is expected to cause a 5.2% contraction in global GDP in 2020 (World Bank 2020).

© The Author(s), under exclusive license to Springer Nature   97
Singapore Pte Ltd. 2021
J. J. Woo, *Capacity-building and Pandemics*,
https://doi.org/10.1007/978-981-15-9453-3_5

While the pandemic has affected economic activity and social life in all countries across the world, policy responses to the pandemic have varied across national contexts. This is in no small part due to differences in levels of capacity and will in different countries.

In this book, I have discussed the various policy capacities that have driven Singapore's response to the Covid-19 pandemic. As I have noted in Chapters 3 and 4, many of the policy capacities that underpinned Singapore's swift response to the pandemic had been established in the aftermath of the 2003 SARS crisis. The two pandemics are therefore deeply interlinked, with past events informing current actions, and Singapore's ability to respond to both pandemics driven by the presence of several key capacities.

Chief among these are the operational capacities that have ensured the continued functioning of Singapore's healthcare system. These include the purpose-built National Centre for Infectious Diseases (NCID) and the large numbers of isolation wards across Singapore's various hospitals, both of which were established in response to Singapore's experience with the SARS crisis. Given Singapore's reputation as a leading medical hub as well as its world-renowned public healthcare system, the presence of such operational capacities should come as little surprise.

Aside from operational capacities, analytical capacities played a significant role in Singapore's ability to rapidly identify and isolated infected persons through contact tracing and quarantine management. Such capacities were bolstered by the presence of a pool of well-trained contact tracers, as well as the ability to mobilise military and police personnel to undertake contact tracing activities. Equally important were the technological tools that were implemented to enhance Singapore's ability to process large amounts of information and quickly detect potential infections.

Certainly, the government's ability to mobilise its operational and analytical capacities depended heavily on its political capacities, which ensured strong political trust among citizens and therefore contributed to a higher level of public compliance with the government's Covid-19 regulations, particularly those related to ensuring social distancing. Effective political communication on the part of key policymakers and political leaders also contributed to political capacity.

Last and by no means least, Singapore's material capacities provided it with the financial resources to fund its policy initiatives and stimulate its economy. The availability of urban-physical infrastructure that could be rapidly adapted and repurposed to house existing and potential Covid-19 patients also helped the Singaporean state to prevent its healthcare system from becoming overwhelmed by the large numbers of Covid-19 cases that would emerge in the early stages of the pandemic.

As I have discussed in the previous chapter, such high levels of infection also allude to shortcomings or deficiencies in analytical capacities that could have prevented the accurate and timely assessment of the infection risks that resided in Singapore's migrant worker dormitories. As I will discuss below, this suggests a need to strengthen those aspects of analytical capacity that can help policymakers detect infection risks at various levels of society as well as identify the causal linkages that may exist across different policy domains and issues.

In any case, this book's discussion of Singapore's ongoing efforts to contain and manage the impacts of the Covid-10 pandemic has shown how important it is for governments to build up and maintain sufficient levels of policy capacity. These capacities can then be quickly mobilised in times of crisis. However, the maintenance of high levels of policy capacity—whether these are analytical, operational, material or political capacities—present policymakers with trade-off between maintaining excess capacity and resource optimisation. I will discuss this trade-off and its implications for public policy theory in the next section.

Beyond NPM: Excess Capacity and Slack

At the heart of this trade-off between slack and optimisation lies a more fundamental debate over the continued relevance of the New Public Management (NPM) approach to public administration and governance. NPM first emerged in the early 1990s, with early proponents of the movement focused on achieving greater efficiency and transparency in public administration through a 'reinvention' of government that involved introducing private sector management practices into the public sector (Aucoin 1990; Osborne and Gaebler 1993; Dunleavy and Hood 1994; Hood 1995).

According to Hood (1995), NPM comprises seven key elements:

- Disaggregation and corporatisation of public organisations into separately managed units.
- Contract-based competitive provision of public services.
- Emphasis on private-sector styles of management.

- Greater stress on discipline and frugality in resource use.
- Visible and hands-on management from the top.
- Formal measurement of performance and success.
- Greater emphasis on output controls.

NPM is therefore focused on ensuring greater accountability and efficiency in public agencies through extensive corporatisation, introducing private sector management practices into public organisations, and the outsourcing of certain policy functions to external contractors. These efforts are fundamentally driven by a need to optimise limited government resources, particularly financial and human resources, without sacrificing policy outcomes.

Yet despite the efficiency gains, scholars have also noted several key limitations of the NPM approach. These include over-bureaucratisation, the dilution of public sector values, internal conflicts within public organisations, and a paradoxical decline in accountability with the fragmentation of public organisations and the involvement of private contractors (O'Flynn 2007; Diefenbach 2009). As I have shown in this book, an over-emphasis on resource optimisation and the market provision of public goods can hinder policymakers' ability to respond to sudden shocks and crises.

Singapore has long been known for its efforts to incorporate NPM practices into its public sector, with the creation of corporatized entities such as Singapore Airlines, Singapore Technologies (ST) Engineering and Singapore Telecommunications (SingTel) indicative of its reliance on market mechanisms and private sector management styles in public service delivery (Haque 2002; Lee and Haque 2006; Sarker 2006; Aoki 2015). However, Singapore's adoption of NPM practices differs from that of other countries in several key ways.

First, the government has retained control over its corporatized entities through the government-owned investment company Temasek Limited, which remains the majority shareholder for most of these entities. Second, several of these 'government-linked companies' also play the role of external contractor for the government, with ST Engineering being a case in point. Not only does ST Engineering provide the Singaporean military with its technology, weapons and ammunitions, it has also during the crisis begun producing face masks for domestic use.

Third, senior public servants often take on leadership positions in the private sector, whether in government-linked companies or in private firms. The result of these three factors has been a significant extent of 'policy co-creation' between public and private organisations, driven by dense networks of relations among organisations and their leadership (Woo 2015, 2016, 2019). Hence despite the incorporation of NPM practices into its public service, Singapore's policy and governance landscape continues to be driven by the government's direction, goals and values.

As I have shown in earlier chapters, this prevalence of government goals and values has manifested in Singapore's tendency to build up and maintain excess capacity. Much of this is no doubt driven by strategic concerns, with the constant threat of military aggression from its regional neighbours driving Singapore to adopt a 'siege mentality' in its governance and diplomacy (Leifer 2000). The most tangible outcome of this 'siege mentality' was the government's efforts to build up a national stockpile of food and medical supplies, ostensibly to prepare the country for an actual military siege.

This stockpile has proven to be useful during the Covid-19 pandemic, with the government able to ensure a steady supply of food and medical supplies, despite disruptions in the regional and global supply chain arising from the pandemic. Aside from the national stockpile, other excess capacity includes urban infrastructure that could be adapted for housing Covid-19 patients, manpower that can be redeployed to pandemic response activities such as contact tracing, and a deep pool of financial reserves that can be mobilised to fund its pandemic response efforts as well as stimulate the economy.

Singapore's experience in combating the Covid-19 pandemic therefore emphasizes the importance of maintaining excess policy capacity or 'slack' as well as the crucial role played by public agencies and government-linked companies in both maintaining and mobilising such excess capacity. This runs counter to the resource optimisation and market mechanisms of public service delivery that is emphasized by NPM. From a public administration perspective, policymakers may need to reassess their approaches to resource optimisation and management, especially with regards to the need to maintain excess capacity in anticipation of future needs.

Such notions of excess capacity or organisational slack have received much attention among scholars of business studies, with these studies emphasizing the importance of slack resources in enhancing organisational performance, innovation and resilience (Moreno et al. 2009; Chen et al. 2013; Stock et al. 2017). Similarly, policymakers and public managers may consider building up excess capacity and organisational slack to ensure the presence of resource and capability buffers that can enhance their crisis response mechanisms.

As I have discussed in Chapter 1 and as the case of Singapore has shown, such excess capacity can help maintain systemic robustness and functionality during a crisis. This presents important policy lessons for governments seeking to emulate Singapore's approach to managing the Covid-19 pandemic.

Policy Implications and Some Caveats

Given its low levels of Covid-19-related fatalities as well as its highly effective contact tracing processes, Singapore's ongoing efforts to manage the impacts of the Covid-19 pandemic have generated much interest among policymakers who are seeking to manage Covid-19 outbreaks in their own countries (Heijmans 2020; Hsu and Tan 2020; Lim 2020; Rogers 2020).

In the rest of this section, I will summarise some of the key policy lessons that can be gleaned from Singapore's experience. At the same time, some caveats may be in order. Given Singapore's unique socio-political context, efforts to emulate the Singaporean approach to managing the Covid-19 pandemic will necessarily require a certain extent of policy adaptation. I will also discuss the limitations and shortcomings that have emerged in Singapore's Covid-19 response, and suggest possible ways in which these can be mitigated.

The key policy lessons that can be drawn from Singapore's Covid-19 response are summarised below:

- The crucial role of contact tracing for identifying and isolating potential Covid-19 cases.

  - Ensuring the availability of trained personnel and clear protocols.

- Calibrated approach reducing social interactions through a 'circuit breaker' rather than a complete lock-down.
- Maintaining excess capacity which can be quickly mobilised during a crisis.

  - These include financial reserves, excess hospital wards, physical-urban infrastructure, and a national stockpile of food and medical supplies.

- Drawing on digital technology to enhance contact tracing and quarantine monitoring processes.

  - Building up a technological ecosystem and infrastructure that can yield useful technological tools and innovations.

- Ensuring public compliance with policies and regulations through effective political communications.

While all of these policy lessons have been discussed to varying extents in the previous chapters, two of these are nonetheless worth reiterating.

First, excess capacity can act as a buffer during a crisis by providing policymakers with a useful set of resources and competencies that can immediately be applied to crisis response efforts. As the case of Singapore has shown, financial resources, the national stockpile, and Singapore's physical-urban infrastructure have all played key roles in ensuring systemic functionality.

Particularly noteworthy is the purpose-built National Centre for Infectious Diseases (NCID). Prior to the Covid-19 pandemic, the 330-bed NCID was largely focused on research and laboratory work, with its isolation wards only coming into full use during the pandemic. The NCID therefore represents a significant investment of financial resources and medical manpower, with 'returns' on these investments only evident during a healthcare crisis.

As I have discussed above, the maintenance of such excess capacities or idle resources runs counter to NPM notions of resource optimisation and cost minimisation. It also goes without saying that the maintenance of a full-scale hospital or the building up of a national stockpile of food and medical supplies requires large amounts of financial resources, as well as the willingness to convert these resources into idle resource that do not generate an immediate return.

Aside from excess capacity, technology has also played a crucial role in Singapore's efforts to contain and manage the Covid-19 pandemic. As I have discussed in previous chapters, the application of artificial intelligence and data analytics to contact tracing has enabled Singapore to collect and analyse large amounts of individual movement and contact data. The informational needs of contact tracing were therefore met by the presence of a sufficiently mature technology ecosystem that could provide the Singapore government with these tools.

Singapore's ongoing efforts to transform itself into a leading smart city has, through no small amount of serendipity, also contributed to its analytical capacity for containing and managing the Covid-19 outbreak. This is also true for other emerging Asian smart cities such as Seoul, which has similarly drawn on cutting edge digital technologies to manage its Covid-19 cases. Unlike many other smart cities however, state actors play a crucial role in Singapore's technology ecosystem, whether in the form of the government's technology agencies or its government-linked technology firms.

The roles of these entities in adapting and developing technological solutions during the SARS and Covid-19 pandemics have been amply discussed in previous chapters, with the Defence Science and Technology Agency's (DSTA) Infrared Fever Scanning System, the Government Technology Agency's (GovTech) TraceTogether App and Singapore Technologies (ST) Engineering's mask production facilities being important cases in point. Aside from government agencies, private technological firms such as Razer have also adapted their production lines to manufacture more face masks.

The technology ecosystem can therefore play an important role in pandemic response, by being a source of technological solutions that can be applied to and/or adapted for crisis management. As cities continue to digitise and governments seek to tap on the emerging technology sector by establishing smart cities, technology will continue to play a major role in future pandemic response efforts. Indeed, the Covid-19 pandemic has already prompted many governments across the world to hasten their urban digitisation efforts, with smart cities seen as potential sources of technological solutions that can immediately be applied to their pandemic response efforts (ABI Research 2020).

Excess capacity and the use of technology are therefore two important policy lessons that can be gleaned from Singapore's Covid-19 response, along with the other lessons listed above. Having said that, any attempts to replicate or emulate these lessons should also take into account Singapore's unique socio-political circumstances.

Specifically, Singapore's limited territorial size and relatively small population has made it easier to enforce laws and regulate citizen behaviour. As a small city-state that has experienced continuous single-Party rule within a majoritarian parliamentary system, laws are also passed much more quickly. Lastly, the communitarian and Confucian political culture that has over the years infused much of Singaporean society also suggests a greater extent of policy compliance among its citizenry.

Certainly, these are factors that may not exist in many countries. The extensive, and often intrusive, state interventions that were implemented may also not be acceptable in other polities. These include social surveillance and control through roving 'safe distancing ambassadors', mandatory orders to wear masks in public, as well as heavy penalties for any transgressions against social distancing rules. Countries seeking to emulate the various policies that Singapore had implemented will therefore need to be aware of these extant underlying factors, the absence of which may hinder successful policy outcomes.

It is also important to note that there have also been shortcomings and limitations in Singapore's pandemic response efforts. These can present useful policy lessons as well.

Despite its high levels of policy capacity and its reputation as a leading medical hub, Singapore was nonetheless afflicted with large numbers of Covid-19 infections. As I have discussed in Chapter 4, much of these arose from large infection clusters within Singapore's migrant worker dormitories, exacerbated by analytical capacity deficiencies that had prevented policymakers from achieving a clearer understanding of the infection risks that existed within these densely-populated and badly-managed dormitories.

Going forward, there will be a need for the Singapore government to strengthen its analytical capacity, particularly in terms of developing better risk assessment processes and enhancing its ground-level understandings of emerging policy issues. As I have alluded to in Chapter 4, closer state-civil society relations can help policymakers to tap on the ground-level knowledge that civil society groups possess.

Aside from analytical capacity, there is also a need to enhance inter-agency coordination as well as develop a deeper understanding of the causal linkages and inter-relations that often exist across different policy domains and issue areas. With regards to Covid-19, this may require closer coordination between the Ministry of Health, which is tasked with leading Singapore's pandemic response efforts, and the Ministry of Manpower, which regulates the operators and owners of migrant worker dormitories.

In order to address the myriad social, economic, political and urban impacts of the Covid-19 pandemic, a 'whole-of-government' approach will be necessary. Comprising ministers from a broad range of policy domain areas, Singapore's Multi-Ministry Taskforce represents a good example of such a whole-of-government approach. Further efforts at entrenching this whole-of-government approach could focus on enhancing cross-functional linkages across different public agencies.

FUTURE DIRECTIONS

While this book has sought to provide a comprehensive understanding of the various policy capacities that have driven Singapore's Covid-19 response, it is by no means the be-all and end-all of Singapore's pandemic response efforts. As at time of writing, Covid-19 infection and fatalities continue to rise across the world. In Singapore, the total number of Covid-19 infections have exceeded 55,000 while the number of fatalities stand at 27.

While much has been written, and more continues to be written, on the epidemiological aspects of the Covid-19 coronavirus, there continues to be a need for more research on the efficacy of policy responses to the pandemic. How have different countries responded to the Covid-19 pandemic? What are the different policy tools and initiatives that have been implemented as part of these responses? What are the determinants of policy success and the causes of policy failure? How can governments build up the capacities and competencies for dealing with future pandemics?

This book, along with the emerging stream of research on policy capacity in Covid-19 response efforts that was discussed in Chapter 2 (Capano 2020; Capano et al. 2020; Hartley and Jarvis 2020; Woo 2020), has sought to take a policy capacity approach to understanding Covid-19 policy responses. In order to develop a better understanding of the policy capacities that can be established to pre-empt future pandemics, there will be a need for further research and theorising on the different policy capacities that have contributed to successful Covid-19 policy responses across different countries.

Aside from policy successes, a deeper focus on the capacity deficiencies that may have led to policy missteps or failures in different countries can also prove instructive for policymakers on what not to do as well as what capacities to build up, in order that similar missteps can be avoided. In any case, policy capacity provides a useful framework for understanding the various resources and competencies that can be built up to pre-empt and address future policy crises.

REFERENCES

ABI Research. (2020). *COVID-19 to Accelerate Adoption of Technology-Enabled Smart Cities Resilience Approaches: Robotics, Digital Twins, and Autonomous Freight* [online]. Available from: https://www.abiresearch.com/press/covid-19-accelerate-adoption-technology-enabled-smart-cities-resilience-approaches-robotics-digital-twins-and-autonomous-freight/. Accessed 14 July 2020.

Aoki, N. (2015). Institutionalization of New Public Management: The Case of Singapore's education system. *Public Management Review, 17*(2), 165–186.

Aucoin, P. (1990). Administrative Reform in Public Management: Paradigms, Principles, Paradoxes and Pendulums. *Governance, 3*(2), 115–137.

Capano, G. (2020). Policy Design and State Capacity in the COVID-19 Emergency in Italy: If You Are Not Prepared for the (Un)expected, You Can Be Only What You Already Are. *Policy and Society, 39*(3), 326–344.

Capano, G., Howlett, M., Jarvis, D. S. L., Ramesh, M., & Goyal, N. (2020). Mobilizing Policy (In)Capacity to Fight COVID-19: Understanding Variations in State Responses. *Policy and Society, 39*(3), 285–308.

Chen, Y.-C., Li, P.-C., & Lin, Y.-H. (2013). How Inter- and Intra-organisational Coordination Affect Product Development Performance: The Role of Slack Resources. *Journal of Business & Industrial Marketing, 28*(2), 125–136.

Diefenbach, T. (2009). New Public Management in Public Sector Organizations: The Dark Sides of Managerialistic 'Enlightenment'. *Public Administration, 87*(4), 892–909.

Dunleavy, P., & Hood, C. (1994). From Old Public Administration to New Public Management. *Public Money & Management, 14*(3), 9–16.

Haque, M. S. (2002). Structures of New Public Management in Malaysia and Singapore: Alternative Views. *The Journal of Comparative Asian Development, 1*(1), 71–86.

Hartley, K., & Jarvis, D. S. L. (2020). Policymaking in a Low-Trust State: Legitimacy, State Capacity, and Responses to COVID-19 in Hong Kong. *Policy and Society, 39*(3), 403–423.

Heijmans, P. J. (2020). *Why Has Singapore Been So Successful in Containing COVID-19 Coronavirus? | World Economic Forum* [online]. World Economic Forum. Available from: https://www.weforum.org/agenda/2020/03/singapore-response-contained-coronavirus-covid19-outbreak/. Accessed 31 March 2020.

Hood, C. (1995). The "New Public Management" in the 1980s: Variations on a Theme. *Accounting, Organizations and Society, 20*(2–3), 93–109.

Hsu, L. Y., & Tan, M.-H. (2020). *What Singapore Can Teach the U.S. About Responding to Covid-19.* STAT.

Lee, E. W. Y., & Haque, M. S. (2006). The New Public Management Reform and Governance in Asian NICs: A Comparison of Hong Kong and Singapore. *Governance, 19*(4), 605–626.

Leifer, M. (2000). *Singapore's Foreign Policy: Coping with Vulnerability*. London: Routledge.

Lim, J. (2020). How Singapore Is Taking On COVID-19 [online]. *Asian Scientist Magazine* | Science, Technology and Medical News Updates from Asia. Available from: https://www.asianscientist.com/2020/04/features/singapore-covid-19-response/. Accessed 25 May 2020.

Moreno, A. R., Fernandez, L. M. M., & Montes, F. J. L. (2009). The Moderating Effect of Slack Resources on the Relation Between Quality Management and Organisational Learning. *International Journal of Production Research, 47*(19), 5501–5523.

O'Flynn, J. (2007). From New Public Management to Public Value: Paradigmatic Change and Managerial Implications. *Australian Journal of Public Administration, 66*(3), 353–366.

Osborne, D., & Gaebler, T. (1993). *Reinventing Government: How the Entrepreneurial Spirit Is Transforming the Public Sector*. New York, NY: Plume.

Rogers, A. (2020). Singapore Was Ready for Covid-19—Other Countries, Take Note | WIRED [online]. *WIRED*. Available from: https://www.wired.com/story/singapore-was-ready-for-covid-19-other-countries-take-note/. Accessed 31 March 2020.

Sarker, A. E. (2006). New Public Management in Developing Countries: An Analysis of Success and Failure with Particular Reference to Singapore and Bangladesh. *International Journal of Public Sector Management, 19*(2), 180–203.

Stock, G., Greis, N., & Fischer, W. (2017). Organisational Slack and New Product Time to Market Performance. *International Journal of Innovation Management, 22*(4), 1850034.

Woo, J. J. (2015). Policy Relations and Policy Subsystems: Financial policy in Hong Kong and Singapore. *International Journal of Public Administration, 38*(8), 553–561.

Woo, J. J. (2016). *Business and Politics in Asia's Key Financial Centres—Hong Kong, Singapore and Shanghai* (1st ed.). Singapore: Springer.

Woo, J. J. (2019). The Politics of Policymaking: Policy Co-creation in Singapore's Financial Sector. *Policy Studies*, 1–18.

Woo, J. J. (2020). Policy Capacity and Singapore's Response to the COVID-19 Pandemic. *Policy and Society*, 1–18.

World Bank. (2020). *The Global Economic Outlook During the COVID-19 Pandemic: A Changed World* [online]. World Bank. Available from: https://www.worldbank.org/en/news/feature/2020/06/08/the-global-economic-outlook-during-the-covid-19-pandemic-a-changed-world. Accessed 21 July 2020.

INDEX

© The Editor(s) (if applicable) and The Author(s), under exclusive   109
license to Springer Nature Singapore Pte Ltd. 2021
J. J. Woo, *Capacity-building and Pandemics*,
https://doi.org/10.1007/978-981-15-9453-3